The
Hungry Soul

Based on a True Story

Jacqueline Knight

ISBN: 1-4196-9469-3
ISBN-13: 9781419694691

Visit www.booksurge.com to order additional copies.

Acknowledgments

I would like to thank Bonnie, Mary D.H. and Lannie for their willingness to read and edit the manuscript, and for their encouragement and support. My gratitude also goes to Holly for voluntarily picking up the torch and taking it upon herself to open the publishing-world doors. I am eternally grateful to my parents, siblings and grandmother for never giving up on me. And finally, thank you to my husband for unconditional love that gave me wings to fly.

"For He satisfies the longing soul,
And fills the hungry soul with goodness."

– Psalms 107:9

Preface

The voice of clairsentience spoke to me late one night as I lay curled in my bed reading. I set the book aside as the inner voice in my head spoke louder and said, "You can write a book." After the hundreds of novels I'd read and many authors I admired, I knew that this was the calling of my soul outwardly expressing a desire that I had kept to myself as I felt it was one attainable only by others.

Three months later, my youngest son started kindergarten and for the first time in seven years I had time to call my own. After I bid my children farewell at the bus stop, I came home, sat at my desk and began to write my first book. I was not under any illusion that the first book would succeed, but firmly believed that through the discipline of a daily writing schedule and continued practice, one day I just might see my dream fulfilled. I gave myself a time frame of ten years to make it into the publishing world. That was in August of 1998.

A year later and with my first book under belt, we decided to make a career move and that meant moving the family across the country. The move proved to be the first of several others and throughout, I continued to write. However, the reality of our financial circumstances and a failing economy began to sink in and I began to grow more and more fearful of our future that was placed in the hands of others. And so I got my real estate license and began selling real estate. I loved the business but still, in the back of my head, that small voice of the soul waited to be acknowledged. In the late evenings, I wrote several more books.

In the summer of 2005, we made our fifth move in six years. Bone-tired and weary, I found myself with a desolate mindset too tired to once again summon the energy needed to jump back into real estate. I wasn't sure either if I should write another book. I wanted to do one or the other, but whatever the decision, I wanted to have a very clear focus and purpose so that I did not spin my wheels. I simply didn't have the energy for that any more.

It was shortly after this last move when I received an unexpected phone call from a dear friend I'd met during our brief Kansas City stint. "I want you to write another book," she said even before I had the chance to express what had been weighing so heavily on my mind. It seemed an odd coincidence and I wondered if this was perhaps a sign.

Lisa insisted that this time my approach should be different, and she encouraged me to write about experiences of the heart.

It didn't take long to realize that there was indeed one topic that was very close to my heart, an issue that had once controlled my every thought, action and decision. It was an issue of the past that I was now far removed from, and also a topic that I chose never to discuss. In fact, there were many within my circle who had no idea that this topic, this illness had once ruled my life.

Over the years and for the most part, I had walked away from my eating disorder. But during those passing years, I witnessed the illness become more and more prevalent within our society. It was impossible not to see the covers of magazines, the talk shows, the media trying to deal with and understand this topic. Having been once locked within its prison, I felt that there was much being left unsaid and that because of this, the aura of mystery continued.

Despite logic insisting that my information could possibly benefit others, I continued to have many reservations. Doubts flooded my thoughts as I silently argued all my reasons for not moving forward. 'Who wants to read about something so dark?' Certainly I was in no hurry to venture back in time, twenty years earlier, to the diseased mindset that once crippled my every thought. No. No one wants to know about that, I insisted. I remained leery and hesitant about writing this particular topic.

But I also felt that there were some truths that needed to be told, truths related to the source of this illness as well as the full scope of mental devastation that occurs once an eating disorder has taken hold. I felt that there were many young women in trouble now who feel that no one understands. It was also impossible to refute the fact that what were once more isolated cases is now a prevalent disease among women and adolescent girls in today's society.

And then I began to realize that the same fears that served to foster and perpetuate the long-ago struggles – fears of embarrassment, humiliation, mockery, ridicule, ineptitude, shame and guilt – were the very same fears holding me back from writing this book.

Once this realization sank in, I began to feel that perhaps this story could help some woman out there, someone who struggles now as I did back then. Whoever this woman may be, this story was written for you.

Valentines Day, 1984
Wt: 133 lbs.

It was a dream that I wish were reality, one that if possible I would willingly trade places with in a seamless exchange from darkness into light. I want to close my eyes again and seep back into the secure softness of illusion that caresses my innermost desire. I do not want to awaken to an ordinary depressing reality, a reality severed from fantasy the minute my eyes open. I want this dream to stay with me, to take over my life, to become a part of who I am, to be my existence. I want it to be real instead of banishing into that unconscious realm where most dreams go, where the evidence is soon forgotten and forever lost. I do not understand why dreams have the ability to torment with the enticement of what can never be.

I lay in my bed with the covers pulled high over my head to ward off the real world, not wanting to go to biology or English class, not wanting to do anything at all. The sun's morning rays beckon through the narrow slits of the drawn mini-blinds, urging me to get up, get out of bed, get dressed, and go to school. I cannot summon the energy to move and I feel more depressed than ever.

I dreamed of Julian, a multi-color, panoramic love story that seemed more real than fiction. He had returned to the shadows of my lost soul. He was back. Julian was back. Julian was back in my life after a two-year absence during which my world had never been the same, one utterly drained by an irreplaceable emptiness in which the heartache had continued to linger. In the dream we are back together, united, having forgiven and forgotten all the bitter actions and ugly words. I am at his side where I belong, and I feel happier than I've ever been before. My shattered world is restored, and once again I feel whole. We sit together and he hugs me. He tells me he loves me. He wants to know what I think. He wants to know how I've been. He *sees* me. He is the only person who has ever truly seen me. I have missed that. I once believed he was my soul mate. I still believe this is true.

Once I realize this deep longing is only a figment of my subconscious desires, I feel more depressed than ever. It seemed so real. I wish it was not a dream. I want to leap inside this fantasy bubble that pops into my slumbering mind and live and breathe its fresh air. I want it to be real.

I have neither seen nor spoken to Julian since before he left for college. Every day I wonder how he is, what he is doing. I think of him constantly. I hear he has a girlfriend.
The thought of him kissing someone else, hugging her, making her feel as special as he once made me feel makes me so sick to my stomach that I cannot bear to think of it. But I do think about it. I think about him all the time. I still miss him.

During these first two years of college, I have not been able to move forward, to progress emotionally. I have remained stranded in time, the observer on the sidelines of life who silently watches as others move forward and carry out their plans while basking in the glow of warmth and the security of purpose.

I have never met anyone else like Julian, and I don't believe someone else like him even exists, someone who is so perfect for me. He was the only guy who ever truly saw me. He could see straight into my soul. I miss him so much. And yet I know he has moved on. Moved on to a different school, a different girlfriend who I've heard through the grapevine is beautiful with long blonde hair and a perfect figure. Of course. I have been so lost without him, so lonely for him, and I have not found a way to deal with the emptiness inside or the sadness that probably should have ended a long time ago. He has moved on, but I haven't managed to do the same.

I still love him, and begin to feel even more depressed with the realization that today is Valentine's Day. I do not want to go to school today and witness anything that has to do with love. I do not want to see all those happy faces, and be reminded of my own emptiness.

My bones are heavy as I try to sit up in bed.

I miss my high school friends who have also all gone their separate ways. I wish we had all stayed together. Why did I ever choose to embark on a separate path? Surely the transition would have been so much easier had I stayed together with my friends. Instead, I insisted on going away alone. Hard-headed me. Back when I felt confident enough to spread my own wings. Couldn't picture myself at the larger state universities. Too big. Instead, I opted for a smaller, more contained environment. It seemed like the minute I split from my friends and tried to make a life on my own, everything turned south, thus beginning a downwards spiral, a descent that only worsened over time. I went from being an A student on honor roll, to a C/ D student with no desire to achieve anything. I don't enjoy school like I once did. There is no motivation to excel at anything. I don't feel any connection whatsoever to that girl I was in high school. I look at those weathered pictures and no longer recognize the girl who smiles back at me. I have failed miserably. I have strayed so far off my path, and I do not know how to find my way back.

There once was a time when I was excited about my life. When I was excited about school, excited about seeing my friends, when I actually set goals to make A's, and made elaborate plans for every party. Now all of that seems many lifetimes ago. How could such a difference occur in a scant two years? There is no longer anything to get excited about, no reason to achieve anything. The spark has been gone for a long time. I don't know where it went. I also don't know why it went away.

I dread the fact that my sophomore year is nearly over. College is half over and I haven't the faintest notion of what to do with my life. I wish I were more like my younger brother who always has a plan, a purpose, and I have no doubt that when he graduates, he will start a company and make his fortune, just like he always said he would. I always admired the fact that he always seemed aware of what his life purpose was, even at the age of ten. I was never like that, much as I always wished I was. He should have been the eldest of our five-sibling gang, the leader, the role model. Not me.

How can I compete with that? Why am I so different? Why can't I be more like him? I am so fearful. What does my future hold? More importantly, how do I extract myself from this current trap?

When I contemplate my future, I see nothing. I have no direction. I do not know where to turn. I do not know which path to follow. The cluelessness only serves to make the past, the warmth of sunny days when I lived at home and relished in the daily friendships of my high school friends, seem that much more enticing. How I wish those days had never ended. I wish I had that time back. I wish I knew who the hell I am, what my purpose is. I hate living like this, merely existing day to day, floating around aimlessly like pollen polluting the atmosphere. This school is costing my parents a fortune and I am fully cognizant of the extent of their sacrifice in order to pay the expensive tuition. I have truly failed them. I have failed them, and I have failed myself.

My thoughts always wander back to Julian, to the past, to a time and place where I long to be. I want to wave a magical wand and revert back in time to when I was in Julian's arms, back when I was happy and felt seen. No more emptiness. No more sadness. No more searching. No more despair. I wish I wish I wish. If I could only, somehow, get back on that track. But I do not know how.

February 15, 1984
Wt: 133 lbs

I feel even worse today. I need to talk to someone. There is only one person who won't laugh. I pick up the phone and dial her long-distance number.

"Mimi?" I say when she picks up the other end. At half past eight, my grandmother has just walked through the doors of the travel agency that she's managed for twenty years.

"Jackie," she answers, her voice happy. She is always happy when I call. In many ways, she has always been the big sister I never had. I know how busy her workload is as she handles arrangements for a large clientele of physicians and that there isn't much free time in her day for idle chit-chat.

However, she is never too busy to talk to me. "What's up with you?" she asks eagerly.

"Not too much," I say, fiddling with the ties of my blue cotton robe while blinking back tears.

She instinctively hears through my disguise, and recognizes the distress hidden behind a mask of coolness. She knows me better than anyone. Sometimes I think she knows me better than myself. "Jackie, what's wrong?" she demands to know.

I pause, not knowing where to begin, not knowing how to release the sadness I've kept bottled-up for so long. Sometimes I feel I will explode from the sadness, that it will eat me alive if it hasn't already.

I am barely able to utter the words. "I had a dream about Julian."

She thinks a minute, trying to recall who I am referring to, what his relationship is to me. It doesn't take long before the faintest of memories recalls within her mind, and she remembers. "I thought he was long gone by now," she says. "Thought you hadn't seen him in years."

I nod to myself. "True," I whisper, barely able to breathe.

"Well, why did you dream about him then? Why after all this time?"

In her usual no-nonsense manner, she has put hammer to nail and articulated precisely the truth. I know it is the truth but still to this day it is a truth I haven't been able to acknowledge. I still cannot admit it is over, that our relationship is history. Tears begin to roll down my face. My vision becomes blurred. I am alone in this apartment and alone in the world, with one life line that waits patiently on the other end of this phone.

"I still miss him," I admit, sensing an uncanny oddness over what seems a massive understatement. "I've missed him this whole time."

"Jackie," she coos soothingly, seeming at a loss for what to say next, how to help. She silently ponders this predicament. "You haven't found anyone since him."

It is not a question for she knows well the answer. Since my going away to college, it is been my grandmother who has inquired about my dating status, wondering aloud why out of so many eligible men, none manage to retain my interest for any length of time. She muses her wonderings aloud, but never makes any negative comments. She has been the one to encourage me to move on, to have fun, to take advantage of the dating pool here at school. *In due time, when you're ready, there's someone out there for you*, she always says. But I never believe her. I don't want anyone else. I only want Julian.

Then she suddenly pieces the rest of the puzzle together. "Yesterday was Valentine's Day and you're missing him even more because of it. Am I right?"

"Yes." The tears continue to roll down my face, down the front of my neck. I wipe them away with the back of my hand, and dab my cheeks with the terry-cloth lapel. Heat flushes my cheeks, my forehead, and my eyes begin to swell. I am so tired. I am so tired. I am so weary from carrying around all this sadness and emptiness. I am so tired of feeling invisible, left out, empty. I am so tired of this constant fatigue.

"Oh, sugar," she says. "I'm so sorry. I'm so sorry. I know it hurts and it hurts a lot, but what can I say?" Her tone is endearing as she tries to comfort.

The mere act of finally admitting this to someone feels better, for she is the only one who understood just how much I loved him, and not once did she ever refute the fact that love can be found at such a tender age. I have not admitted this to anyone until today, until this conversation when this weight is finally released. I have not said anything because of the sadness and confusion, feeling too dazed, too lost, not willing to admit the truth – that our relationship is long over. I have not been able to let loose his memory and move on with my life. My heart was ripped apart and I never knew how to pick up the pieces. I did not know how to replace the emptiness or how to remove the sadness of losing someone I so dearly loved. I have held myself back because I do not know how to move forward. I do not know the necessary steps to take that will carry me back into the emboldened rays of the sun and shed light on a promising path that stretches ahead rather than remaining stuck on this dusty dry crossroad that continues to look backward.

"I want him back," I say. "I want things to be the way they used to be." There it is, the declaration that, until this moment, I did not realize is what I truly want. I want my old life back. I want the happiness of the past to return. I want the love and security of yesterday, and that includes a full restoration of my relationship with Julian.

Somehow I managed to lose all of this as the pieces of a broken heart continued to fall apart, leaving traces scattered throughout the blinded course of the past two years. Everything has fallen apart since I went away. Somehow I feel that Julian is the key to regaining the lost happiness, a long narrow trail strewn with sadness and loneliness that I need to part from. I believe this is the key that will turn my life around, put it back on track, a new course filled with love, purpose, happiness and a new sense of self-worth.

"There you go," she cheers, summoning all the enthusiasm she can muster. "That's the old Jackie that I know. So what's to say you can't have him back? What's to say he doesn't want the same thing?"

I ponder her question curiously, as it is something I hadn't before considered because I naturally assumed that because he has a girlfriend, he's happy and is life is fulfilled and .... There are too many and's and but's attached to this long list of possibilities.

Still, the doubts are there. "He wouldn't be interested in me," I say.

"And why not?" she asks.

"Because I'm fat," I say.

"You are not fat," she says adamantly. "You are not fat and I won't have you saying that. I won't allow you to put yourself down." If only she knew what a pro I am at putting myself down. Surely this is the one thing at which I do excel.

Feeling suddenly self-conscious, I draw the openings of my robe closer to my chest. I am hidden within its large size, the long sleeves, its floor-length. I do feel fat. Twenty pounds have collectively gathered onto my thighs and gut since freshman year. Twenty pounds that cause my clothes to fit tightly, jeans to zip with difficulty, the hollows underneath my cheekbones to disappear. I am embarrassed by the extra weight, embarrassed at how I look, embarrassed by how it makes me feel. But that embarrassment by itself has seemed to somehow join forces with the other cumbersome issues that are always present. Combined, they form a monstrous mountain of weights, problems that seem impossible to figure out. Too many emotions are simultaneously convened into a mountain too high to climb. Its peaks and crevices stretch so far into the horizon that I don't know which stone to examine or attempt to budge first. And so I don't do anything at all. I have felt helpless to do anything about it. I haven't known where to begin. Somebody show me what to do!

"Mimi, you saw me at Christmas … all that weight I've put on…"

"So you put on a few pounds," she ventures. "So what. All freshmen gain weight. It's because of all those heavy starches they serve in the cafeteria to feed the athletes. There's no way to prevent it. So what. Big deal."

"The equivalent of eighty Quarter Pounders is a big deal," I say. "I look horrible and nobody in their right mind would dare show any interest in me while I look this way."

"I guess when you put it that way," she chuckles. "But you don't look horrible and plenty of guys ask you out. It's been your choice to turn down everyone who's asked. But if you feel that way, then do something about it. Fix yourself up. Start taking care of yourself again. Lose the weight if you must. Twenty pounds isn't such a big deal to lose."

"I don't know how to lose the weight," I say, and once again I feel shamed at knowing just how many things I do not know.

"Diet, exercise, the same way everyone else loses weight. Go get yourself a book at the store and read up. You're resourceful."

As I listen to her, the tears begin to dry. I begin to feel the faint twinges of newfound hope, of untested promise begin to pour through the blood in my veins. It seems like forever when I have felt any hope or promise whatsoever. These visions and ideals are, in my mind, reserved for others, and certainly not for me. I begin to think that perhaps this is not just a far-fetched dream, but rather, a definite possibility that could transform into a realized goal if I devise a specific plan of action and then follow-through accordingly. If I could indeed realize my dream of a restored relationship with Julian, I know that somehow, some way, I can summon the willpower to stick to a weight-loss plan.

Stirrings of hope begin to pump energetically through my veins, and energy that has remained dormant for so long begins to filter through. Could I do it? Could I lose the weight? Could I fix myself up? With renewed hope, I wonder if I can do it even though I feel as if I haven't been able to accomplish much of anything in these recent years.

These thoughts are interrupted again by my grandmother who is not yet finished. "Jackie, I want you to listen to me. You're smart. Damn smart. And you're a beautiful girl with big blue eyes and long brunette hair. You need to look in the mirror and see yourself the way I see you, the way everyone else sees you. For whatever reason, you haven't been able to do that in a very long time. You need to take a good long look in the mirror and also realize that you are capable of accomplishing anything."

Her declarations seem foreign, as if she is referring to someone else. Me capable? What have I ever accomplished? All I have done while at college is fail miserably, fail in every aspect of my life. What have I ever accomplished? Nothing. However, what is true is the fact that I have been lost for a very long time. I veered far from a path that I have not been able to find my way back to. How could this have occurred so suddenly and within such a short period of time? Still, what makes me think I can accomplish anything as I have no record of recent achievements to speak of.

"You got accepted into college, didn't you?" Mimi counters.

In my mind the accomplishment seems too small to be considered of any meaningful value. The much anticipated acceptance letter followed immediately by the sudden cliff dive. A collapse that defied explanation.

She continues. "Forget about all that. What you need now is a new sense of accomplishment."

"How?" I ask.

"Well, she muses, "let me think a minute. Okay, here, I've got it. Do your parents know about your grades?" She refers to my two D's and three C minuses.

"No," I say.

"Well then, that's the first thing. It is now the middle of February which leaves plenty of time for improvement by the end of the semester. Can you do this?"

I consider the possibility and realize this is certainly within my ability. I've done it before and I can do it again. It would mean really buckling down, long evenings spent at the library, no more missed classes, but yes, it can be done. "I guess so," I say, realizing how unconvincing I must sound.

"Good," she says. "Now on to the next issue – Julian. Will you see him this summer?"

My stomach lurches at the possibility, for I feel certain that with a little luck and the right timing, chances are very high that I will bump into him somewhere. Although Houston is a large city, in many ways it is a very small town. Last summer I avoided any possibility of running into him anywhere. I did not want him to see me wearing all this extra weight, to witness the evidence of my downhill slide.

"Probably," I say, knowing the chances are very real and that somehow I will find a way to see him, but only after I trim down and pull myself back together.

I glance at the mirror at the far end of the hall, and shudder at my reflection. I do not like what I see. Hair's a mess. Too short. Color's bad. And this weight. Oh my god, this weight!

I begin to wonder if I can indeed lose the weight, take better care of myself, improve my grades. I wonder if all of this is possible within a short time frame of three months. New pressures begin to mount like before, only this time I do not mind so much because my desire to attain these goals is of utmost importance. Yes, it is possible. It is possible but only if I begin today. There is just enough time to turn my situation around, just enough time to accomplish this before returning home, the new me, at the end of the semester. I begin to feel better.

February 16, 1984
Wt: 133 lbs

Jill likes rocky road as much as me. But somehow my roommate has managed to maintain her cute petite figure. After classes, she asks if I want to take a break and go to the Creamery for a cone before heading off to the library to study.

We refer to ice cream as a cone the same way we call any soft drink a Coke. However, it is never just a mere cone that we order but rather a hot fudge sundae or a banana split, something with plenty of calories. Somehow calling it a cone makes it seem acceptable, less of an indulgence, and therefore guilt-free.

"Sure," I say.

The small store is chilly and goosebumps form onto my arms and legs. Brightly colored posters adorn the walls and picture windows with photographs of mouth-watering desserts. Jill and I order, and then take our ice cream to a quiet table in the corner. She has already indulged in her two scoops of chocolate. I ordered my usual: a sundae with one scoop of pralines & cream, hot fudge and extra cherries. We do not say much; our friendship is comfortable even in silence.

Jill takes another bite while I spoon my first into my mouth. Warm chocolate fills my palate, delicious fudge that is soothing, comforting. It slides down my throat and I savor the aftertaste. I think about my conversation with my grandmother and how grateful I am that she was there to answer the call. I don't know what I would have done if she hadn't been there. I think about how much better I feel after our conversation, and the new sense of purpose I now have. The previous tiredness and sadness are replaced with a new sense of rejuvenation and strength. I do not feel the same dread for tomorrow, the dread of going to classes alone, sitting in the back seat alone, waiting for graded papers to be returned to me with D's and C's. That is all in the past for now I have much work ahead and not very much time in which to accomplish my new goals.

Twelve weeks remain to achieve these goals, and this realization begins to sink in as to just how short a time period this really is. Before I know it, May will be here and I'll head home for the summer. Three short months to improve my grades to the pre-college A's, and three short months to knock off all this weight. Twenty pounds to lose in just three months. Twenty pounds. Twenty pounds in ninety days. As I idly stir the dish of melting ice cream, the magnitude of this daunting task begins to sink in. I continue stirring the fudge that now grows colder. Twenty pounds in ninety days.

Mentally calculating, I figure it equates to approximately 1.6 pounds per week. One point six pounds per week to reach my destination, to the freedom that lies ahead, freedom from this sadness and overwhelmed mental state I've been living under. Yes, of course I can do it, I think hesitantly, willing it to be attainable, wanting it to be within my grasp. I do not know how, but somehow I'll find a way. I haven't the foggiest clue how to lose the weight but if others have done it, so can I. The sundae has long since lost its rounded shape and has melted low into the dish, a gooey blackened mixture of sugar and cherries that looks neither enticing nor edible.

Jill's eyes now waver from the oncoming traffic on Mockingbird Lane to the uneaten dish before me. "Eat up," she insists. "We need to get to the library."

One-point-six pounds per week. The phrase repeats itself over and over in my mind as it grudgingly eeks out a newfound stake of willpower and determination within a mind that for so long has lacked either of these traits. *One-point-six-pounds per week* continues to reverberate along the membranes of brain cells that long for a new awakening, a jump-start to re-charge and re-energize. *One-point-six-pounds per week* cries out louder and more fierce, demanding to be heard, refusing to be ignored. *One-point-six-pounds per week* beats a steady rhythm to the deep drum sounds of the jungle where an order is first created, then repeated, in monotone, as it develops into a new mantra from which to live by, a sacred calling by which the linen shadows of the forest listen and silently obey.

One-point-six-pounds per week is the only hope I have to cling to at this point. It is the only hope I have of removing myself from this depressed state, from the constant unhappiness that weighs so heavily. It is the link that will bring me back to the earlier state of happiness, to the days filled with belly laughter and many, many friends. For me, it is the difference between death and life.

I want the old me back. I want to be that happy girl again. No, I don't want to be *that* girl again. I want to be a much improved version: better, thinner, smarter, livelier. I do not want to live so sad and depressed any longer. Now that I think about it, I don't even think I want to come back to this school where I so obviously do not fit in.

However, everything depends on one thing. I'm not worried about the grades for I know those can be easily improved.

It's the weight. Knocking the weight off. Twenty pounds is all that is required. The bridge to my new freedom. I don't know how it can be done but, as I stare into the melting dish of sad and abandoned ice cream, I realize that eating any more of *that* will only prevent me from accomplishing my goals. I'll never be able to lose the weight if I eat this ice cream. Even a single bite could cause the entire plan to fold. It may bring some short-term satisfaction but that's about all. Another bite of that ice cream will place yet another barrier from my new destiny that awaits with open arms. I will see this weight gone. I will not remain stuck in this idle emptiness forever. Never. If I dabble into even the tiniest bite, my situation will never change, and I'll be stuck in this black hole of sadness and emptiness forever.

I stare into the bowl of ice cream through new eyes of awareness. It no longer represents sweetness and short-term satisfaction, symbols of summer and celebration. No. Now its meaning is entirely different. It is a symbol, a symbol of choice, one that will either keep me harbored within this empty reservoir or serve to turn the corner and begin anew.

"Are you not feeling well?" Jill asks. She is not used to seeing me forego dessert.

I do not feel I can explain. There is too much to explain, too many factors now fully assembled into one gigantic ball of determination set within my brain. How can I begin to explain for it would mean going back too far in time and explaining everything. The story is too long, too long and too painful to remember if only because it is what has led me to my current state, a condition I abhor, a mindset I detest. This girl that is me who has struggled so much over the past two years is not who I want to be in the next two years, or ever. As the weight begins to discard, she will slowly disappear and in her place will emerge someone new.

Armed with newfound determination, I stand, carry the dampened container to the trashcan, and toss away its entirety. The color spectrum of browns and black easily slides from the plastic container onto a mass of discarded paper napkins. The debris of white paper then slowly begins to absorb the blackened mixture, its hue and texture gradually changing shape and color as it transforms from white to beige until all is finally settled and lost in a sea of dark cocoa.

February 17, 1984
Wt: 133 lbs

Someone once said that I pursued things wholeheartedly. That, of course, was several years ago, before my heart splintered and split into a million tiny fragments. I never knew that one incident can alter an entire life, that sunlight can be eclipsed so easily, that the road can become invisible once your footing goes off-track.

I purchase two pocket-sized books. The first is a calorie glossary of every type of food imaginable, including fast food, along with the caloric value of each. I need to learn this, and not just learn it, but memorize every word. It must be ingrained into memory. I must instinctively know what I am feeding my pie-hole as this is the key to finding my way back again to the light.

The second book pertains to diets and gives a sample menu of each day, in all — thirty days worth. I browse through the latter but do not find what I am looking for. I want to know exactly how many calories need be consumed in order to lose one-point-six-pounds per week. Exactly, and not a single calorie over that limit.

I did not eat breakfast this morning. Lunch consists of chicken salad and a cup of cream of mushroom soup. Salad for dinner. I suspect the salad is not really as low-calorie as I anticipated. Cheese, turkey, ham, croutons, bacon bits, salad dressing. Can one really lose weight eating all these things?

Physically I feel no different today than I did yesterday. Still a bit lethargic. Studied a lot. Made an outline of what I need to review since January. There is much catching-up to do. *One-point-six pounds per week.* The mantra chants its rhythm, urging me to conform, to adhere to the plan. Can I do it? I started today, or at least I think I did. Still, it seems an awfully long way from here to there.

February 23, 1984
Wt: 133 lbs.

I ate a salad every day for the past week. It doesn't really fill me up, but there's something enjoyable about the time required to eat a salad properly. One bite after another. Chewing the lettuce. It has a rhythm, a slow rhythm that is strangely comforting. I like salads except for the fact that I am hungry two hours later.

I'm afraid to weigh myself. I'm afraid that I've eaten the exact lunch and dinner for a week straight, a 'diet' in my mind, and that I haven't lost any weight. What if I continued this diet of chicken salad for lunch followed by a salad for dinner – for three months, and ended the semester the same big fat pig I was at the beginning? I cannot allow this to happen. I will do anything to prevent this from occurring. Nothing will stand in the way of achieving my goals.

February 25, 1984
Wt: 132 lbs.

I bought a scale and keep it hidden underneath my bed. So far I've lost one pound. A single pound closer to my goal, to the freedom that awaits me. And yet, it's also one pound shy from that girl I am trying to forget, to lose, to wash away, to make disappear. The distance between moving forward and that of moving backwards is exactly the same and rests in the precise measure of a mere sixteen ounces. I need to continue. I must continue. I must focus. I must lose the weight. If I've lost one pound, then surely I can lose two more.

Salad dressing contains more calories than all the other ingredients combined. From now on, I will only use low-calorie dressing.

March 1, 1984
Weight: 131 lbs.

Another pound gone, but I can't stand the fact that the scales continue to exceed the 130 mark. My jeans aren't quite as snug, but there is still a long way to go. There will be no rest until all the weight is lost.

I am worried about returning home this summer. I am worried about how I fit in with my family, or rather, the fact that I seem so out of place there and don't belong. I wish I could be the big sister that my siblings deserve, someone they could look up to and feel proud of, not this ridiculous nineteen-year-old who doesn't have a clue who she is or what she wants to be when she grows up.

I wear a mask that feigns strength. However, beneath this plastic façade there is no strength to be found. I have been in the process of falling apart for years. When I should have been walking forward, I actually did the reverse.

College in nearly half over and I haven't the faintest notion what I want to do with my life, what career I want to pursue. I feel quite certain that if any of my siblings were standing in my shoes right now they would know exactly what they wanted. Surely they would have a plan.

I wish I were more like my brother who has had his life plan mapped out by the age of ten. His plan never wavers and follows a sequential path of graduating from college, starting a company, making millions of dollars by the time he reaches thirty, retiring, and then perhaps getting married. My brother has always possessed the gift of seeing possibilities in situations where others do not. When the city experienced a drought during the summer of 1976, forcing local jurisdiction to outlaw lawn-watering between the hours of seven a.m. and midnight, my then eleven-year-old brother turned this to his advantage by forming a single-employee enterprise, himself, and servicing the necessary lawn maintenance while all the neighbors snored into the wee hours. He made nearly nine hundred bucks, a fortune at the time, especially to a kid.

Richard has always had a plan, and there's no doubt in my mind that one day when he graduates, he will indeed start a company and make his fortune. He'll probably live in a big Mediterranean-style home that has one of those swimming pools where water pours forth from the open jaws of concrete lion heads.

I have always been able to see his potential. I have always had the ability to see the potential in others. I can look at others and immediately recognize their many capabilities, their endless possibilities, and their sure successes. But it is not the same when I view myself, my self-worth always compared to others who are, no doubt, better.

How can I compete with that? My brother has always had a plan. And now, two years before I am to theoretically embark upon the 'real world', I haven't a clue, not a single clue of what to do with my life.

My time is running out and I am afraid. I am afraid all the time. The clock is ticking and I wish there were some way to make it stop. *Tick tock, tick tock,* it taunts, drawing me nearer and nearer to that point of finality that is supposed to be met with acceptance and certainty and purpose. *Tick tock, tick tock,* it teases, mocking me because I do not have a plan and do not know which path to follow. *Tick tock, tick tock,* it chants as the rest of the world continues to move forward while I remain benched at the sidelines of purgatory, unable to participate fully among the laughter of the living.

I wish I were more like my sisters who, like my brother, would no doubt have a plan by now. How disappointed they must be in me for I am nothing like them. Leslie, about to graduate from high school, the over-achiever, the natural athlete, voted most popular, and winner of the prestigious and VERITAS award, the highest award given at her school. Leslie who has the personality of a dozen girls, who can charm and befriend a rattlesnake and make it lick icing from the palm of her hand.

Then there's Abigail, the family beauty, a beauty that belies an intelligence that makes her a natural storyteller, the best I've ever known. Abigail the cheerleader, Abigail on the Homecoming Court. And then there's Daniel. The funny one. Daniel who has more friends than anyone I've ever known. Daniel who will never be lonely.

And then there's me, the big failure. Big. Huge big. If only they realized just what a complete and utter failure I am. How can I even begin to compete with all they have accomplished, with all they will accomplish in the future?

March 5, 1984
Weight: 130 lbs.

A Cosmopolitan article explains how running causes faster weight loss. I know nothing about running. I have never been athletic nor have I ever participated in any sport. I read that running and jogging knocks off weight faster than any other form of exercise. It not only causes more rapid weight loss, but it also keeps it off. I will try running

March 9, 1984
Weight: 130 lbs.

Bought a pair of burgundy New Balance's with extra shock protection. Want to find out if I can jog if for no other reason than to knock more weight off, and faster. Time is ticking and the deadline looms just a short distance away. There are a few girls who jog at the track in the afternoon. They are thin and don't look like they even need the exercise. Why are they out there? Could I ever look like that?

March 19, 1984
Weight: 126 lbs.

Night continues to fall early in the late winter months, creating an eerie hush across the rows of stately oak trees and the long winding corridors of the campus grounds. The university track sets behind the freshman dorms. Orange stadium lights illuminate an oval running pad that provides a cushion underneath my feet. Several runners, mainly female students and residents from the adjoining neighborhood, are usually out this time of the evening. They have become familiar figures darting in the distance of the dark shadows.

I stretch my legs, bending over to touch my toes, stretching my calf muscles. My attire is not designer-appropriate like that of the other runners. I wear a pair of old shorts and a worn t-shirt bearing an emerald green emblem for melon liqueur. I head around the track, slowly at first. Two laps quickly pass and I realize that I actually enjoy running. The other joggers, who are in much better shape than me, have already passed me several times. Each round in passing, they manage a sideways tilt of the head and a hand lifted in mid-air, a friendly gesture to their fellow joggers. This is how I am now perceived – as a fellow jogger.

I prefer to run at night, in the dark, with the icy winter freeze pressing against my face. Even surrounded by the other joggers, there is a certain anonymity when running at night for while the others may see a form struggling to run in the shadows of their familiar trail, they cannot truly see me. They cannot see my ruddy, sweaty face beneath my cap. Nor can they read my expression or guess my thoughts. They know not my name, my history or my reasons for being here. I am completely anonymous. In my anonymous state, I can be anyone I want to be.

It is the same for the other joggers. I can barely make out their shapes and forms, thin shapes and pale colors of pink and yellow running attire as they make their stealth moves against the silence of the settled blackness. Likewise, their faces and the details of their expressions remain concealed within the safety of the darkness. While I may see them, I cannot truly see them.

I continue moving forward, willing my legs to continue their strides as they pound one-two-three-four against the softened asphalt in a comfortable mode that is neither too strenuous nor too easy. I check my Swatch often, knowing that every ten minutes represents another mile completed. My goal is to run two miles a day. So far, mission accomplished.

The evening air is quiet as the birds gather back in their nests and the cold keeps the sane indoors. There is much to look at even among the shadows. Across the way, the baseball field is empty as the spring players have finished their afternoon practice. In the backdrop lies the shadows of the dorms, symmetrical triangles and rectangles that form a mini-village against that of the surrounding atmosphere. One by one, trickles of lights pop onto the sky's nighttime canvas as students retire to their rooms after supper. They are inside where the air is warm, and I am out here on the track where I am free.

Without actually hearing the inside noise, I sense the endless chaos of several hundred girls all laughing crying, whining, screaming, chatting. From experience I can sense it. I can feel the chaos from the outside looking in, and I am glad to be out here in the blackened silence with only the sounds of my footprints padding against the cushioned blacktop and the steadiness of my own breathing. I can sense the warmth that lies within the dorms. Orange flickers of fluorescent lighting. I can feel the warmth that lies within. Warmth tempered with the noise and chaos that never ceases. Warmth that sings out to me across the wide back lawn to the track as it beckons for me to re-enter into its safety zone. It is the barrier between me and them.

I like being out here in the peace and quiet and night air. I like that no one can see my face, and that I have alone-time to think, away from the constant chaos of the dorm that is not unlike that of the chaos inside my head. I like that jogging gives me a sense of rest and peace. I like being anonymous. I like the fact that I can run two miles. If I can just hold on to this latest small sense of accomplishment, hopefully I will able to accomplish much more. I want to accomplish *something* with my life. I'm just not sure what.

April 25, 1984
Weight: 118 lbs.

My boss at the bistro pulls me aside after the lunch rush. "You're disappearing before my very eyes," he says, and his tone feels doubled-edged, as if he's paying me a compliment yet accusing me of something else. "You've lost a ton of weight, and you look good. But enough's enough. You don't need to lose any more weight."

I do not tell him that I've lost fifteen pounds, although I do outwardly acknowledge that I am three shy from my goal. Tugging at his moustache, he shakes his head in disbelief. "Girls these days – all of you – everyone wants to be thin. You're thin enough. Look at your clothes hanging baggy on you now."

It's true, clothes fit much more loosely, and I now require a belt for my pants. I feel a sense of pride that he's noticed the weight loss, a sense of pride that I'm still firmly set on track to reaching my goal. But I'm not about to quit now.

He continues. "You used to eat my chicken salad. You used to come in here every afternoon and pour yourself a cup of my homemade cream of mushroom soup. Now you come in here and eat nothing. I offer to fix you a plate myself but you refuse. What's the matter? You don't like my cooking anymore?" He is a wonderful chef, the reason his restaurant is so successful.

I tell him I'm very busy, that I often now take my lunch before I get to work. I assure him that his chicken salad is the tastiest in the world. Even that doesn't seem to appease him. He doesn't believe me.

What I don't tell him is that once I realized meals at the bistro contained too many calories, I decided to delete them from my menu. There is no way to reach my goals by eating chicken salad and rich, creamy soup every day. I don't tell him that his gourmet food has been replaced with a plate of green beans that equates to one hundred calories. I don't tell him because I know he wouldn't understand. Every day as I prepare to leave his shop, he offers to prepare a to-go plate for me. "For later," he says. But I always refuse the offer.

I think I have worried him, and for that I feel badly. But I will not quit dieting just because he believes I've reached a healthy weight and look good. He doesn't know a thing about me. He doesn't understand that everything, everything hinges upon this weight loss. I cannot quit now. This new me is beginning to emerge and people are starting to take notice. Slowly, parts of the past are discarded. My shape has changed entirely. I am slimmer. My legs are strong from running. For the first time in a very long time, it feels as if I am in control, back in the driver's seat instead of being the silent passenger in cargo. I cannot let go of this. I fear if I get lazy and cheat, all the weight will return. Even one tiny taste of forbidden foods has the potential to reverse all that has been achieved. In an instant I could be back where I started, back at square one, staring into the mirror at the lost girl who knows no direction.

April 26, 1984
Wt: 118 lbs.

Joel phoned. His fraternity wants me to be a Little Sister.

Surely there has been some mistake, I wonder aloud.

No, Joel says. The vote was unanimous.

I can't help but think this must be a joke. Pick me? Little Sisters are always the cutest and most popular girls. I am none of these things. I am nothing, a nobody. Although I move with the masses, the steady crowds of co-eds marching to and from classes, at all times I feel invisible. And though I may speak and laugh and at time feign the illusion of gaiety, inside I feel locked away and trapped. I feel separated from the rest of the world, from the co-eds on campus, by an invisible wall, a colorless, odorless shield that allows me to see out but prevents others from seeing in.

I fail to see what this fraternity thinks they see, the reason for their enthusiasm to make me a permanent fixture in their crazy, funny brotherhood. I do not see what they see, and I fear accepting their invitation. I fear their disappointment should they realize who I truly am. I fear their disappointment should they realize the real me, the girl I see when I look into the mirror. How I would love to join their crazy, funny world and let go of these mental weights that continue to bog me down. I want to say yes but my fears will not allow it. *Not yet*, the fears say, *not until you have reached perfection by accomplishing your goals.* I am so close. And so I continue to stand idle at the same crossroad as before, fully realizing that my saying yes could possibly help in moving me from this stranded posture.

But the fears are too powerful. They say no. And so I thank Joel but tell him I cannot accept. He does not understand. Of course he doesn't understand. How could he ever understand? I feel horrible for having disappointed him and for hurting his feelings.

April 27, 1984
Wt: 118 lbs.

Perhaps my preoccupation with my grades and my weight has gotten a little carried away. Since the diet began, I have pulled way back from my friends who don't understand why I don't want to order pizza at midnight, why I don't want to go to bars and drink with them, why I don't go to fraternity parties, why I don't want to have fun. I don't know why either. I just know that I *don't want to.* I am laser-focused on this diet, and all else just gets in the way.

Friends now say things like "I wish I could lose weight as fast you," and "I wish I had your willpower." They tell me how thin I am, how good I look. Inside I blush but there's still something nagging away at me, something that questions their sincerity. I look at myself in the mirror and see that although I am three pounds shy of my initial goal, there is still so much fat hanging onto my middle, my thighs, my face. I still don't feel good enough. This near-end result still leaves much to be desired.

Final exams are in three weeks and then I'm done here. I do not want to return to this school. I never did fit in here and I realize that most of that is my own fault, for not trying harder, for not having a better attitude, for automatically judging everyone, assuming they were judging me, negatively of course, first. I made a mess of my life here, spun downwards in a cycle that doesn't seem to have one distinct starting point of destruction. I don't know why this happened. I don't understand why I never felt like I fit in. I want to finish losing the weight and then start somewhere new. I want to start my new life over in a new setting, a different environment.

April 28, 1984
Wt: 117 lbs.

I phone my brother. He's not in so I talk with his roommate who I feel very close to. When he asks how I am doing, I am honest. I tell him about the weight loss, about the running, about the self-imposed distancing away from friends and all social events. I tell him that since I went away to college, I have felt like I am drowning. I tell him I do not want to return although I am having second thoughts, doubting myself on this decision.

He tells me he has decided not to return to his university either, and that in a similar way he and I are in the same boat, facing the same decision. He says, "Jackie, you have to ask yourself, are these the friends I want to have for the rest of my life? And if the answer is no then you need to leave and find the right place for you."

When I hang up the phone, my decision is made. I will not return. I need to start fresh, somewhere new. I must leave this rubbished mind behind and finally pick up the pieces to start again.

May 1, 1984
Wt: 115 lbs.

I am always hungry. Hunger is always there, a foe that whispers in my ears, *"You're starving, you're hungry, eat something, eat something, eat anything, eat....."*

I am always hungry, always thinking of my next meal, counting down the hours until I can have that next apple for breakfast, or a heaping plate of green beans for lunch, or a salad for dinner. I am always hungry, and the constant rumblings in my belly are temporarily staved off with diet sodas whose carbonation is filling.

I am hungry in the evenings when I make my way to the track to run. Running always makes the hunger go away, at least temporarily. But by the time the last mile is completed and I come home, shower, change and head off to the library, the hunger returns and once again I attempt to stave it away with another diet drink.

I realize now that my diet may not be as private as I had thought. People are starting to notice exactly what it is that I do eat. Every day at lunch is the same. I enter the cafeteria line, grab a tray and silverware, and move along the slow progression. Pointing to the steaming silver tin of green beans, I pause and wait for the Cafeteria Lady to dish out another plateful. It is the same lunch I had yesterday, and the day before, the same as last week and last month. It is the only food I ever order in the cafeteria.

The Cafeteria Lady looks as if she's worked there a hundred years. She is perky at the beginning of the year but by the end of second semester, she just looks exhausted, ready for the school year to end and her summer to begin. A thin net covers her gray hair, wisps of loosened white tendrils framing her pale wrinkled cheeks. This time she does not so readily give in to my request. She pauses, places a hand against her hip, and takes a long look at me, longer than she's ever looked at me before. It is if this time she truly sees me, sees straight into the insides of my being. I am uncomfortable in the spotlight of her discerning stare. It is a look that demands explanation, an explanation I will not offer for truly, I could offer no other explanation other than the fact that I am just on a simple diet. Surely even she can tell how much weight I had gained, how much I still need to lose. I pretend not to notice her long demanding gaze.

The line waits. I feel the impatience of the other girls behind me whose chatter and laughter have died down as they now curiously peek out from the linear formation to see what's holding everything up. I am horrified by their stares and again pretend not to notice. Deep in my gut forms the beginning sickening feeling of utter panic. My face flushes a vivid crimson hue, and at that moment my only desire is to be invisible. If I cannot be invisible then I wish I could escape from the demanding stare of the Cafeteria Lady, from the curiosity of the other girls. Silent sirens blare in my head, begging for an escape but there is none, and this would only draw more attention. I feel helpless, and now angry at the Cafeteria Lady who has created all of this unwanted attention now directed at me. Nothing makes me feel worse than unwanted attention. It socks me with raw fear, creating a sickening pit in my gut.

I look at the Cafeteria Lady, silently praying that she'll just hurry up and dish out the damn beans, give me my plate and leave me alone.

There is a pleading in her watery gray eyes as she continues to stare firmly into mine. A pleading for me to eat something else, something other than the beans. She tries to mask her disapproval. Does she also attempt to silently discern my new ways? No matter how hard she might try, she cannot begin to fathom what's in my mind.

She sighs, ladles two big scoops of beans onto a clean plate, and then hands it to me. But before I can reach it, she draws it back to herself, and then reaches again for the ladle. Muttering to herself, she says, "If that's all she's going to eat, I might as well give her more." She pours a third helping onto my plate.

May 5, 1984
Wt: 111 lbs

I am always surrounded by people yet I feel so alone, a ghost that walks among the crowds, unseen, unheard. This thought crosses my mind each time I enter the school cafeteria. Seated with my plate of green before me, I gaze across the dining hall that is filled with pretty girls and it is not the first time I think to myself, "What am I doing here?" I do not fit in. I know it. I feel it always. Not that a single soul here has ever said or done anything to cause me to feel this way. It is just the way I feel. Absolutely inferior. This is a beauty pageant. I've not been in this cafeteria when the atmosphere was not positively bubbly. Bubbly personalities. But bubbly is never how I feel inside.

I reach for my first bite of beans and start chewing. Slowly. Slow chewing to make the meal last. I add salt and pepper to provide for some taste.

There are so many pretty girls in this room. I admire all the pretty clothes, the perfect hair, the perfect bodies. How did I end up in a school where I so obviously do not fit in? I compare myself to each one of them and always come up short on the measuring stick. There is no way I can compete. How could I ever compete among this class of young women? I don't even dare dream it is possible. My extreme shyness prevents me from making more friends than I have.

I feel I am being judged at all times, that while they are smiling and talking to me, inwardly they are taking mental notations of a long list of defects. Everything seems like a competition. Is it just here or was this always the case? Wasn't there competition in high school too? To be the funniest or the prettiest or the smartest? I do not remember it being so. I only recall the laughter. Maybe it was indeed competitive, maybe I'm just being naïve.

I never expected to feel like this when I left home. I never thought that I would be in a place where I felt invisible, a nothing. Nothing to give, nothing to share, nothing worthy of being noticed, nothing worthy of friendship. I do not recall ever feeling like this. And yet, the instant I tell myself this, I know it isn't true. In fact, nothing could be further from the truth. It is my secret, a secret I have kept to myself, a secret I have never told anyone. To tell the secret would only expose myself to further humiliation and embarrassment.

It is my secret. One that I've never felt the slightest compulsion to reveal. It is something I walked away from and forgot about. Or so I thought. I could never reveal this secret to my friends and take the chance that they would view me in a different light, see me through the eyes of the others from a time long ago. If I did admit this secret, they just might see the truth: that I was not worthy of friendship, that I was funny-looking, that my clothes were dated and laughable, that my face and body were ugly, that I was awful, that no one would ever like me, that no one would ever like me, that no one would ever like me.

It is a secret of the past. And yet, here I am six years later and those old feelings have reappeared. How do I make them disappear? Maybe if *I* disappeared, the feelings will also vanish. Despite my empty stomach, I no longer feel hungry. I feel silently panicked, edgy in my chair, suddenly unnerved by the possible *What-If's*. What if the remainder of my college years were spent as they were in grade school, always the nobody, believing I was a nothing? I am panicked because I see how easily a repetition of the past could unfold before my very eyes. It could happen if I let it, if I lost control, if I skipped a beat and allowed any of the past to re-enter and pollute my world. The fear that it could happen again is paralyzing. And yet it is this fear that takes over every ounce of reserve within my soul, an emotional force that springs to life, overpowering everything else with a steely resolve, declaring that never ever will I allow *that*, my secret, to happen again.

There is also another secret, one that I will never reveal to a living soul. Nobody knows. Nobody will ever know. I never think about it, and most of the time I forget that it is even there. At least that's what I tell myself.

No matter what I have to do, where I have to go, what I must change, how little I must eat, this thing I do know: that I will not allow the past to repeat itself. I would rather be dead than go through that again.

May 18, 1984
Wt: 111 lbs.

My mother meets me on the driveway, her arms wide open. She is followed by Fatty, an eighteen-year-old Siamese hellion, and Growly, a rescued feral cat with notched ears and lips. She seems happy to see me although I feel hesitant to trust this as I am fully aware of just how difficult a teenager I have been. Hopefully those days are behind us.

At age forty-five, my mother looks a decade younger. She wears minimal makeup; in fact her entire outward appearance is one of simplicity as evidenced by a pair of faded blue jeans and cotton peach t-shirt. She hugs me and it feels real as warmth radiates from her strong pianists' hands. Five inches taller than her, I feel like Godzilla standing at her side. I have never had the petite frame that my sisters also share with her. Lucky girls.

She says let's unload the bags and get settled back in. She has kept my room exactly the way it was before I left. Nothing has changed, she says. She takes a second look at me and tells me I look good, that she can't believe all the weight I've lost. She says, "You sure did that fast, honey." She says let's go to lunch tomorrow, just the two of us. It will give us a chance to catch up.

May 19, 1984
Wt: 110 lbs.

The lunch crowd has already formed at Criley's Cafeteria. The aroma of baked corn and hot apple pie wafts throughout the parking lot. I do not tell my mother just how much the smell of combined food bothers me. The mixture of fried fish and fried chicken and baked apples and creamed corn. There is a Daily Specials blackboard with the words printed in chalk: Vegetable of the Day: Macaroni and Cheese. I smile to myself and my mother gets the joke as well. We begin to laugh. My mother comments again on my weight loss. She did not realize I had even been on a diet. How did I do it, she wants to know. How did I do it? How did I do it so fast? Exactly how much did I lose?

I proudly answer her questions, but I do not want the interrogation to continue. It seems as if she has difficulty comprehending what I have to say, the daily routine self-imposed for the past three months. My mother has had five children and still weighs what she did in high school. She has never had a weight problem. She has never been heavy, not even by a few pounds.

I feel funny explaining my diet to her, as if I am exposing myself to my previous failure, the failure of gaining weight in the first place.

Not only did I not tell my parents about my diet, but I have yet to tell them about my decision to not return to Dallas. I don't know how I'll explain it. They'll freak. My mother will be the most upset of all. I still remember the pride in her eyes that first morning of leaving when she told me, "You're the first person on my side of the family to go to college." Yet another invisible bar in which to measure up.

We find an open table in the crowded room and set our trays on a Formica table for two. My mother has a plate of collard greens, fried okra and black-eyed peas. She drinks water. She eyes my plate: a side of peaches and a double helping of green beans. She does not say anything.

The air-conditioning is turned way down and I spread a napkin across my lap like a blanket to keep warm. I wish I had a sweater. I hate being cold. So many things tumble through my mind that I can't place a finger on exactly one particular thing. Although the diet has been achieved, the fact remains that I do not feel better about myself. In fact, I feel more worried and anxious than ever before. It's as if my mind is a washing machine stuffed with clothes, constantly circling and whirling in a spin cycle that never stops. It won't stop. It never does. My mind never stops. As a result, fatigue sets in and I am tired all the time.

I want to enjoy this lunch with my mother because our times alone are rare. In fact, I can't recall the last time just the two of us sat down together at a restaurant. She looks rested, happy, young. She is my mother and I love her.

Elderly ladies wearing pink uniforms, crisp white aprons, opaque panty hose and white Keds push aluminum carts up and down the aisles. "Coffee? Tea?" they say. Having skipped breakfast, my hunger has finally caught up with me. I think, looking at my plate of peaches and beans, that there is no way this amount of food will suffice for the hunger I feel inside.

Hunger. My best friend for the past three months. Hunger, my best friend who guarantees a future filled with many successes. Hunger is my best friend, the impetus that will bring the boyfriend back and make the sadness and stillness disappear. Hunger, who never allows me to forget he is there. Hunger, the price to pay in order to discard all traces of a girl I can no longer tolerate.

My mother bows her head in prayer. I avoid looking around, knowing how this simple act of reverence never fails to stir surrounding interest. I rest my hands in my lap. Out of the corner of my eye, I see two elderly women smile to one another when they understand what my mother is doing. Then, as silently as she began, my mother's eyes re-open and she unfolds the paper napkin and places the silverware on the table. She seems relaxed and genuinely pleased to be spending this time alone with me. We enjoy several minutes of silence.

Between bites, she tells me again how wonderful I look. I blush with pride and thank her. She says, "You must have really worked hard to lose all that weight. I'm proud of you."

I act like it was no big deal, that it was just a passing thing.

The story of the past three months begins to unfold in my mind, a documentary re-enacting itself starting with the conversation with my grandmother, the dumping of the ice cream sundae, the education regarding diet and calorie counting, the steady elimination of calories, the wondering whether I could run a lap around the track that ultimately led to running three miles a day. The mental cameras continue to roll as I recall the daily weighing on a scale kept hidden underneath my bed, waking up every morning with only one thing on my mind which was: when I step on the scale, will I have lost any more weight? The film continues with the hurt glances from my friends as I gradually pulled away from every last one of them, their repeated attempts to try to include me in their activities, the concerned look of the Cafeteria Lady as she was forced to scoop out yet another plate of green beans, the gray clouds that began to settle within my mind and wouldn't go away, the compulsion to lose more weight to attain what was and is, in my mind, perfection. The film continues with worries over my future, worries that lead to an overwhelming anxiety that won't go away. Anxieties that I try to run from each evening on the track.

The mental pictures conclude with this moment where I am now seated with my mother. Only it's not the ending I perceived three months ago when I envisioned happiness and peace. I feel no peace, only worry and fear. Everything around me is gray. Gray clouds stay in my head and won't go away. This was not the ending I perceived and I do not understand why. Something is wrong and I do not know what it is. From outer appearances I should be one of those that happy-go-lucky girls at school, shouldn't I? But on the inside, I feel anything but that. My head, the washing machine, whirls non-stop on spin cycle. Which item of clothing should I sort first – the shirt or the pants? That's how it feels. All are jumbled into one monstrous ball of weights within my head and I can't sort anything out. It continues to weigh heavily, and I just wish it would go away.

My mother smiles at me. She cannot see the tumbling and tossing in my head, even now as I feel it more than ever. I smile back.

"Have you thought about what you're going to do this summer?" she asks.

I tell her next week I'll make some phone calls, try to get my old jobs back lifeguarding at the pool. Those things I'm not worried about.

"By the way," my mother says, "your daddy and I rented a beach house the first two weeks in August."

"Can we afford it?" I ask. They haven't taken a vacation since the kids started college.

"Daddy says we can," she says. "I just hope you can be with us for the entire two weeks. Think you can work it into your schedule?"

I ponder this for a moment, not the scheduling, but rather the actual two weeks spent with my family. I think about how difficult it will be to adhere to a strict diet amongst a crowd of seven who eat often and heartily despite their skinny frames. It is one thing to stay on a diet in my solitude, but quite another to adhere to this discipline among others who are not a part of it, and who would unquestionably raise a unison of eyebrows at the way I carefully prepare a lettuce and tomato salad. Suddenly I feel very nervous.

"What is it?" my mother asks, witnessing a change in my demeanor that she does not understand. "What's wrong?"

"Nothing. Just thinking is all."

She continues. We want you to be with us because before we all know it, summer will be over and it will be time for you to return to school."

There it is. How will I tell them?

I have difficulty finding the words, knowing full well how disappointed they'll be. In the back of my mind I hear her words the morning I first went away to school. *You're the first one in my family to ever go away to college, to get a degree.* She and my dad were so proud of the fact that I was admitted into a prestigious school, you would have thought I'd received an acceptance letter from Harvard. This will kill them.

"About going back," I begin. "I'm not."

"You're not what?"

"Going back."

"You're not going back to college?" There is alarm in her voice and her mood immediately changes. She sets her fork on the linoleum and earnestly studies my face.

"No. I mean yes. I mean yes I'm going back to college, but no I'm not going back to Dallas."

She looks at me incredulously. She cannot believe what she is hearing. She does not want to hear what I have to say.

I try backpedaling. "Mom, I know that school is costing you and dad a fortune." *A fortune they don't have.* "And I know all the sacrifices you're making to put me there." *Sacrifices I am not worthy of.* "Richard is in Austin. Leslie goes off to College Station this fall. Abigail and Daniel are in private schools...." There is no short-term end in sight for the financial stresses that lie ahead.

She places a hand on the table, trying to grasp an underlying cause, some reason to explain this sudden change. "Do not worry about the money," she says adamantly. "You're father and I have gone this far. We will continue. We want you to get a good education. The best education." Her voice is soft yet filled with strength. She means it. She will not back down. I can tell this won't be easy. But there is no way I can return to where I have been.

How can I begin to explain to her my true reasons for not wanting to return? That her first-born is a complete failure, the object of ridicule from years of torment in grade school. I'm not the cheerleader or the beauty queen like my youngest sister. Nor am I the most popular and class president like my middle sister. How can I tell her that I can't compete against them or anyone else, that I never measure up to anything, that I never feel like I can accomplish anything, and that I'm always *always* afraid of everything? How can I even begin to explain the sadness I felt after leaving high school, the heartache of missing Julian, the sense that my heyday is behind me and that nothing is in front of me except for what is now made possible because of the weight loss?

How can I begin to explain how much I miss all my old friends, how much I miss laughing all day, every day, or about the mind that tumbles without ceasing except during the brief nighttime reveries brought about by merciful sleep. How can I explain that which I cannot physically see – the gray clouds that suddenly converged from nowhere and grabbed hold of my mind and won't let go? Or about how terrified I am of everything – of failure, of what to do with my life, of ruining it the way I've ruined these past two years.

The goal has not only been achieved, but exceeded. However, the terrors have not gone away. I am still afraid. For whatever reasons, my fears have only become that much more magnified over the past several months. I cannot see past tomorrow or next year. I do not know what lies beyond the dark curtain that envelops me. But I fear whatever it is. I fear a return to Dallas and being once again enveloped in that same darkness for another two years. The washing machine continues to spin and whirl through a cycle that never completes its course. The machine won't quit. It never stops.

How can I begin to explain any of this? It sounds crazy, I know. All I know is that I cannot ever return.

My mother sits patiently, trying to understand, wanting to get her point across, but trying to remain open to what I have to say. "It's just two more years," she says. "Two more years until you graduate and go out into the world."

I do not want to hear this. *Out into the world.* My mind fights this reality. I do not want to go out into the world. I can't even function in the one in which I dwell let alone consider moving into a totally separate solar system. The world is not ready for me either. I am not ready. To go out into the world and do what?

Fear. Fear begins to set in again. Fear. My second best friend who vies for my attention against my first best friend, the entity named Hunger.

I shake my head in silence. I cannot make her understand. I cannot even make myself understand because what I feel inside does not make any sense. I spoon the peaches around and around the plate in an endless circular cycle. The peaches rotate but go nowhere outside the confines of the china rim, just like my life. Despite an empty belly, I am no longer hungry. For the first time in three months, I feel no hunger.

I feel utterly drained. Drained of nothing. Nothingness, which is what I am. I am so tired.

"Jackie," she begins.

I place an elbow on the table, and set a hand against my cheek. The weight of tiredness from my heavy head releases into a supportive hand. My face feels hot. I feel alone and forget that I am seated in a public restaurant. I feel so alone. All this weight inside my head. All this weight. It is too much weight to carry around for another day. Too much weight. The spin cycle won't stop. The gray clouds won't go away. Before I finish whispering the words *I can't,* tears begin to well in my eyes, and droplets of salty moisture sprinkle onto the table top. I feel utterly helpless. There is nowhere to go, nowhere to turn. My shoulders begin to stiffen and I begin to tremble. In silence, the tears continue to pour forth.

My mother remains seated in silence but I can sense her growing alarm. She does not know what to do, how to react, how to comfort me, how to begin to understand. She is alarmed by what she sees, this unexpected pouring of defeated tears that is so unlike the daughter she thinks I am. She begins to realize there is much more behind the statements than what I have let on, than what I am willing to say, than what I am capable of admitting. She realizes there is something terribly, horribly wrong, drastically off. She remains seated, a silent witness to the pain I feel inside.

I feel terrible now for having ruined our rare time together. Terrible that I have ruined her day. Terrible that I have wrecked her dreams. Terrible that I cannot reach out to her any more than she can reach out to me.

Through the haze of tears, I see her worried countenance. She is more alarmed than I've ever seen her. And then, just then, during that brief moment as she looks into my eyes and I into hers, our souls meet in unison and lock together. I feel as if she truly captures a glimpse into the inner recesses of the hell in which I've been living, the whole messy interior that I've tried so hard to keep hidden from everyone, that part of me that is so confused and embarrassed that I don't know where to turn. She captures a glimmer of something so dark and sinister, something that has no name, something she does not know what to call. However, what she does know, what she realizes with her whole heart, is that whatever it is, *it is real*.

"All right," she says, stretching an arm across the table to hold my hand. "Whatever it is, it's going to be all right. It's going to be okay." Her voice is reassuring, warm like I remember from my youth. "If you don't want to go back there, then it's decided."

Gratitude. Despair. Gratitude. Utter despair. Grateful that she somehow was able to see through the façade of masks in which I've been trying so desperately to hide.

"You don't have to go back. If that's not the place for you, there's always another school." She tries to sound reassuring, tries to ease my tears, tries to do whatever she can think of to relieve me of a burden that neither of us understands.

Thank God she somehow saw it. I don't know what I would have done if she hadn't. I don't know what I would have done if my parents would force me to return to that school. For one brief moment, her heart saw into mine. It saw the pain, and in that instant it made its decision.

July 25, 1984
Wt: 106 lbs.

Only three weeks remain of summer and I have spent the entirety of it alone. I have not seen much of my old friends who, for good reason, have grown tired of asking me to do things with them just to have me always respond with my standard reply of 'No thanks.' I miss them even though there have been plenty of opportunities to spend time with them. I miss them but they do not believe this because I now come across as so stand-offish.

The only friend I do spend time with is Kristen. She doesn't make me feel nervous or self-conscious. She is funny. She likes to talk about everything, and I like to listen to her. I can't explain why, but Kristen feels safe to be around. I can't explain what's safe and what isn't, but what I do know is that the path of safety is narrow and not found just anywhere. Kristen does not ask about my unwillingness to hang out with the old group of friends although no doubt she's curious. She does not ask or pry into my new eating habits or inquire about my weight, nor does she judge me. My sense is that she knows something is wrong but figures if and when I want to talk about it, I will. Otherwise, she respects the unseen, invisible boundaries and accepts our friendship for what it is.

I have not seen Julian either although I think I have caught several glimpses of his car on the road. I miss him still, but am glad I haven't run into him. I wouldn't know what to say, how to react. I am still not presentable enough to resume a relationship with him. I am not presentable enough because I am not good enough, and honestly, I don't know if I ever will be.

The gray clouds have worsened over the hot, humid months, and fatigue overwhelms my mind and body every hour of every day. I feel tired when I awaken in the morning, and exhausted when I get home from work. In the early evening as I lace the ties of my running shoes, a mental summons of sheer will is the only thing that stirs the energy needed to run yet another three miles. The long treks along the pavement are accomplished only through what little adrenaline remains. And yet, once the feet are set to pavement, the grayness in my head suddenly disappears, mercifully leaving my brain for the half hour or so it takes to run. However, barely an hour after the exercise is finished, the somber clouds begin to return and re-group in my head. Their sojourn is ever brief.

This summer has not been what I imagined. I guess I had envisioned one happy evening after another spent with all my old friends, laughing, clowning around, playing juvenile pranks and hanging out at the beach. But this has not been the case, again strictly of my own choosing, my own self-imposed exile. Even living in this big house has changed, as I now feel isolated among my brothers and sisters who don't seem to share the same concerns of my parents regarding my weight. They jokingly assign the nicknames Anna, for anorexia, and Ethi, for starving Ethiopian. The nicknames disappear the instant my mother overhears and commands them, in no uncertain doubt that they are never ever ever, not ever to use those names again.

The fact that they joke suggests that they view me as thin. But I don't feel thin. Not even after all the weight I've lost. I feel heavy, weighed down, overwhelmed. Surely I can lose even more weight. Maybe that will help to finally alleviate the clouds, to take away the anxiety, the worries, the fears. I wish I were as thin as they think I am. They think I am someone I am not. It is as if they see someone else, someone other than me. I feel trapped inside, a small speck that nobody can see, a sliver that no one can touch. A small speck that can not seem to float out of its trap.

I have spun myself into a solitary cocoon. However, I would rather be in my cocoon than *out there*. It is much more comfortable inside this web of faux silk where no one can see me or judge me, where I am alone in the food that I can control. Food is the single aspect in my life over which I possess complete control. It is comforting but it is also lonely. Loneliness is another new companion. Loneliness, fear, hunger. The triplets. The companions who have replaced all of my old friends. And yet, aren't these the choices I have made? Surely yes, even if it is the only choice I feel I have.

Still, this way of life doesn't seem right for a girl my age. Nothing about this roller- coaster of grayness and emptiness seems normal. Surely this isn't how a twenty-year-old female is supposed to live her life, an existence devoid of hope. I know this is not the way it is supposed to be. Where did I go wrong? And yet I feel there are no other choices. I wish I knew what my choices were, if in fact there are any.

July 27, 1984
Wt: 105 lbs.

The real world awaits my arrival just two short years ahead in the distant future. It is a thought so terrifying I can hardly bear to give it serious consideration or ponder any of my choices. It is a thought so horrific that I want to crawl into a tiny ball and crawl back into the womb where all is safe and where there are no fears.

What choices do I have? Do I have any choices?

Why do others seem to so eagerly anticipate their futures while I, on the other hand, remain stuck in my cocoon, afraid to venture out even in the safety of night to catch a breath of fresh air? What do they know that I do not? What do they see that I can't? What key do they possess that I lack? Why does everything seem so easy for others and so difficult for me?

What choices do I have?

I don't feel I was ever given many choices, and I wish this had not been the case. I wish I had been given the choice to leave my grade school and attend another. Instead I kept silent, never telling my parents about the horror. I endured the horror and remained silent, assuming that no one would understand, that no one would take my side. I endured the horror back then by building my first cocoon and living within its sticky walls until the long-awaited day of eighth-grade graduation finally arrived. At that point I walked out of my cocoon for good. I walked out of its sealed walls, neither grateful for the protection it had provided nor sentimental about the duration throughout which it had sustained me. I left that cocoon for good, or so I thought.

I wish I had felt that I had choices other than to automatically accept the belief that an adult male could hurt a child and get away with it.

I wish I'd been given a choice to feel the way I did: angry, hurt, helpless, hopeless, lost, fearful, worried. I wish I had had the choice to acknowledge the rage, the fury that took over and consumed an innocent little girl.

I wish, I wish, I wish, I wish. Choices I wish I'd been given in the past.

Now I look into my future and still I do not know what choices there could be for me. I wish there was another choice other than that which seems automatically assumed for my future – that I will one day marry and that a man will take care of me. No one seems to understand how helpless and hopeless that makes me feel – that my entire fate rests in the hands of someone I have not even met.

I envy my brothers for I feel they have been given a world filled with choices for the single reason that they are born male. The world expects them to march out as soldiers and conquerors. They are expected to build and grow and achieve and succeed. The world does not expect them to shove their dreams and goals in the back of a closet and instead assume the reigns of someone else's expectations.

I wish there were choices that involved potential outcomes that weren't negative – like my running – I run because if I do not, the pounds will pile back on. I fear that if I do not run, I'll gain all the weight back within a week. I do not run because I enjoy it. I run because it keeps the weight at bay and temporarily abates the gray clouds that clog my thoughts.

I wish that all my choices were not grounded in fear. I wish I had choices based on the premise of promise rather than the fear of what will occur if I do not choose this path or that path.

I do not know what my choices are therefore I do not know where to turn or in which direction to walk. In the meantime my head continues to spin with anxieties. Shadows of fear lurk behind my every move and thought. I do not know how to escape the tossing and turning that constantly shakes and rattles the insides of my head, or the gray clouds that appeared at some point I do not recall and then worsened in darkness and size to the point where I can barely stand the weight any longer. I can barely breathe beneath the gray clouds.

July 28, 1984
Wt: 105 lbs.

The guilt I carry only seems to make this situation even worse.

I realize that I am not supposed to feel the way that I do, and that none of it makes sense. I realize that I'm damn lucky compared to many others. I am lucky to live in a home where my parents love me, where my brothers and sisters love me, where my grandparents live across the street and also love me. I realize I am lucky to have food on the table, a nice home in a nice neighborhood, a car to drive, and the good fortune to go to college without having to pay for it myself. I live in a pretty family where everyone is pretty, where everyone has an interesting, intelligent, funny, witty personality. I am lucky to have a father who's worked hard to help build a business with a good reputation, and that because of this my family enjoys all the perks that go along with a solid name and reputation. I realize I am fortunate because all of these things are nothing that I contributed to or helped build or did anything to deserve. I realize I got very lucky by being born into this family. I realize how lucky I am that I was not born a female in a third world country where women are treated with less respect than the filthy dogs that run along the dusty roads. I realize that I am lucky to have a father who always treats me with respect, who opens doors for me, who carefully interviews my dates.

The reality of my fortunate circumstances only adds to the guilt. How could I have made such a mess of my life, to be so directionless, so unfocused, so clueless, so filled with a sense of helplessness...all things that do not line up with what is expected of my privileged life.

July 31, 1984
Wt: 105 lbs.

In the early morning, my grandmother telephones. "I just got to work," she says, "but I've been thinking about something for a week now. Thinking and worrying about it, wondering whether or not I should tell you."

"Spit it out," I say.

I hear the hesitance in her voice as she tries to carefully choose her words. "Well," she reluctantly continues, and then pauses again. "I promised that I wouldn't say anything." Her end becomes quiet.

"What is it?" I demand.

"You promise not to repeat it or get mad at the person who told me?"

"I promise," I vow. My curiosity is now fully peaked.

"It's about Julian."

Immediately, my heart leaps as the image of his face, that handsome smile, fills my mind. Warmth and happiness flood my bones, as well as a faint ray of hope. How I miss him. After all this time, I still miss him. "What about Julian?" I ask.

"Something happened last week," she continues. "After you left one morning for work."

I mentally summarize the events of the prior week, unable to recall any specific incident that stands out as unusual.

"What exactly are you referring to?" I ask.

"Your sister says he asked her out."

Dullness overcomes me. Dullness, numbness. Defeat. Fatigue. Utter fatigue. This is not happening. I cannot move. My legs turn to lead, heavy, cementing my feet onto the floor. My shoulders and arms are as heavy as concrete, and it doesn't take long before their weight feels even two tons heavier. I am dead inside.

I say nothing, breathing heavily, taking in uncontrolled deep rasps of air. I cannot get enough air into my lungs. My chest begins to hurt. I cannot get any air into my chest. My legs are oak logs that will not budge. My arm, so heavy now, can barely contain the weight of this phone against my ear. Dead. I am dead inside. There is nothing left. Any hope that once is now gone. How could he do that to me? How could he do this to me? How could he?

I feel dead inside. Speechless. Remote. Far away. Alone on a boat without an oar that is sailing out into the tide with the waves. This is not happening. This cannot be happening. This was not the plan. This was not supposed to be the outcome of the weight loss. This doesn't figure into any part of my plan. How can this be happening?

And my family has known about this for a week. No one has told me of this. They must all be laughing behind my back. I feel so humiliated. I cannot believe he did this to me, knowing full well how I have always felt about him.

Rage. Rage that cannot be acknowledged. Rage towards him. There is no rage towards my sister for I know she is an innocent party. She would never do anything to harm me.

My grandmother continues. "Your sister is beside herself. She is so upset about this, Jackie. She hasn't slept for a week because she's so upset. She knows how you feel about him and she also believes that if you find out, you'll hate her. She made me promise not to tell you and I gave her my word. But after thinking about it, letting it settle for a week, I realized that she's not the one who should feel badly about this. She's carrying around all this guilt, plus she's worried sick about you, and she doesn't want you to find out because she's afraid of what you'll do. She's afraid of what it will trigger. She's afraid that you'll eat even less and run more. She's afraid that you'll despise her."

There are no words for how I feel. I feel my sister's pain. And I am sorry that she spent the last week in such misery because of me. Because of him. I feel her pain, and my own pain stands in her company under the same umbrella. The pain. And the rage.

"I'm not trying to purposefully go behind your sister's back but I really feel you should know what kind of person you're pinning all your hopes on."

I try to find enough air to fill my lungs. I am drowning. I cannot breathe. I lean against the countertop for support. This news was the last thing I ever needed to hear. Not now, not ever. It can't be true, and yet, I know in the back of my mind that it is indeed true, even without having to confirm it with my sister. I know it is true.

I feel no anger whatsoever towards my sister. How could any young man *not* want to ask her out after they take one look at her? I know that my sister did nothing to invite this. I know my sister would never intentionally hurt me.

"You're not mad that I told you, are you honey?" Mimi asks with deep concern.

"No, I'm glad you did." And that I truly mean.

We hang up and I remain immoveable as lead. I have dissolved out of my body, out of my life, rocketed straight into the gray hazy cloud that hangs overhead, straight into the cloud that I hope will take me away from all of this for good. What good was any of the dieting? What was the point? What good was the dumb diet when the outcome will always be the same: failure, embarrassment, ridicule, mockery, shame? This will never end.

August 15, 1984
Wt. 100 lbs.

He is dead to me, just like those other things from the past that caused so much pain. I never think about them as they are locked away and cannot touch me. I am mad, probably angrier than I am willing to admit. But more than that – humiliated. Have I brought this upon myself? What

64

can be done to prevent the past from recurring? I can't believe I have wasted the past two years thinking about him so much. Time that could have been spent building rather than pining. But I never could see ahead into the future, let alone the next unseen day. How did I get so stuck?

I will park his memory into that sealed container within my mind that stores all the other memories I choose to forget. From this point on, he will have no bearing in my life. I have wasted so much time longing for what would never be, and pinned hopes on what I knew in my heart was structurally unsound. That is over now.

August 21, 1984
Wt: 98 lbs.

My mother suggests that I transfer to the University of Texas. "All your friends are in Austin, she says. Maybe you'll enjoy it more there," she says.

I explain that I'd rather stay at home, attend a local university. In fact, I have decided to enroll at the university here in town. I will live at home.

"But you won't know a soul," she says as trepidation registers in her voice. She does not want the past experience to repeat itself.

"That's okay," I say. "I'll meet people."

And so this morning, armed with my transcript, I go to register. Standing in front of me in the long line is a young man, the most handsome young man I've ever seen. He is tall and brunette, with perfect bone structure, piercing blue eyes, and a glowing tan. He wears an un-tucked, un-ironed button-down. I cannot take my eyes off of him, and I realize I am not alone in my assessment as every other girl in line also stares in his direction.

I do not know his name, nor do I speak to him as he is absorbed in a conversation with an older man standing next to him. I merely stand back and admire, as one admires a fine painting. If this is any indication of the rest of the male population at this school, I think I will like it here.

After the registration process is complete I walk to the university bookstore, and buy what I need. I sit on a bench with my sack of new textbooks. A girl sits next to me, a stranger to me, like everyone else. I am still thinking about that handsome guy from registration and secretly hope that he will be in one of my classes.

The girl sets down her heavy bag, sighs and leans back in a long stretch. "So," she smiles at me, "what do you think so far? By the way, I'm Lee Ann." She eagerly extends a hand.

"I think the guys at this school must be very good-looking," I say, shaking her hand.

"Oh?"

"I saw the most beautiful version of the male species I've ever seen before," I admit.

"And who might that be?"

I describe his face, his height, his build. She seems to recognize the description and her face suddenly transforms into one of quizzical expression.

"And he also seems quite intelligent," I add.

Then she asks if he was wearing a button-down shirt, and begins to describe its un-ironed pale blue shade, his outdoorsy appearance. Apparently she knows exactly to whom I refer.

As I begin to nod, *yes, yes, yes that's him, that's the one,* her demeanor takes on an even more astonished reflection, and I know she is holding something back. She stops, and then after a second of pure silence, bursts into laughter, a howling so loud it fills the narrow aisles of the bustling store. Every nook and cranny hears her uproar and hooting as she hollers out loud trying to tell me something but unable to because she is so overcome with hysterics.

"I know exactly who you're referring to," she gasps. "and he's no student either."

"A teacher then?"

She cannot contain herself. "You could say that."

"What?"

"He's a priest."

August 27, 1984
Wt: 99 lbs.

I don't know what to do, and I despise myself for my inability to handle anything the right way. Now I have hurt someone I have always loved, not in the way I thought I loved Julian, but loved nonetheless. People don't always fall into some tidy little category, a stereotype that takes the guess work out of a relationship's determinant factor. And this is how it is with Patrick.

When we first met, me at the age of thirteen and he at fourteen, I immediately sensed that I had known him my whole life. This, of course, is nonsense, even though at the time I could swear to the strangest flicker of recognition that seemed as if we had always known each other. At that first introduction, I saw that same recognition in his eyes, and even though this remained unspoken, it was the basis of an instant bond that established an immediate friendship. I knew that he would always be a part of my life.

Although he lives nearby, we do not see each other often. But now although we'll be attending different universities in the same city, and I had been secretly looking forward to seeing him more often. After tonight, though, I know this will never be the case. I really blew it this time.

Patrick took me to a dance at his school. I was so excited to see him, so excited to spend time with him. It was the first I've been that excited in I don't know how long. Patrick arrived at my door like a long lost friend whom I could not stop hugging. It is a friendship that I haven't been able to describe other than to say it is as if we've been close for many lifetimes, and had not tonight's ordeal occurred, we would have remained close throughout this lifetime. No matter how much time elapses between our visits, it is always as if we saw each other just yesterday.

The early part of the evening began wonderfully, with both of us laughing. There was much to catch up on, much to talk about, and really, we were just happy and content being together.

But as quickly as he reappeared into my life, that's how quickly the gray clouds returned to my head. We were seated in a Mexican restaurant, drinking margaritas and eating tacos. Well actually, he was eating tacos and I was sipping margaritas. He didn't say a word about my not eating.

As I sat across the table from him, I thought to myself how handsome he was, how funny and smart he always was. He was always one of my favorites, of anybody. I thought about how dumb I had been by not spending more time with him when time had been so readily available. While he talks, his khaki-green eyes twinkle, and I know that he feels the same way about me as I do about him. It has always been this way. And I took that for granted. I allowed some dumb delusion of the past to skew my outlook and haze over what was real, what was right in front of me.

But the gray clouds were never far away. As we sat and laughed and enjoyed each other's company, I could feel those gray clouds begin to force their way back into my mind, and fog my thoughts just as surely as if I was standing outdoors in an bare Kansas field watching the weather patterns take a sudden turn, as huge cumulous clouds unexpectedly roll in and tornadoes begin to drop from the sky, destroying everything in their path.

One minute I was fine and the next I was not. Without warning, the gray clouds reappeared and forced a clamp down onto my brain, once again dragging me back into the isolation of its invisible prison. No matter how hard I try, I cannot will them away, and they only worsen in power and magnitude with each passing minute that I sit in the restaurant. The bold Southwest colors of the hanging piñatas, country flags, tropical drinks and mosaic tiled tables transform into black and white as I revert further and further inwards to that mental prison that beckons my return. I no longer hear the strumming guitars or the Spanish tunes sung by the band of mariachi players. Patrick's mouth moves as he continues to speak but I do not hear any words. As the prison walls further envelop me, I no longer hear anything. The mental walk down the long isolated corridors within my mind continues until once again I find myself in a place locked far away from the outside world.

Patrick cannot help but notice the sudden change in my demeanor. He looks concerned. He asks if I'm all right. I reply that I'm fine. But I'm anything but fine. I know these clouds too well. I know the prison they form, the prison from which there is no escape. I know they won't go away. I know how they ruin everything. They remove all life, and leave me stranded in a deserted cemetery.

I have now fully lost my concentration and connection to the outside world. I am unable to focus on anything Patrick says. It is if he is speaking and I hear nonsensical utterances that make no sense. Words fade in and out, but nothing makes sense. They are static waves undecipherable to the ears. I cannot smile either. I am drowning in these clouds.

Patrick takes me to the dance but I cannot smile. I cannot laugh. I find little to say. I am so far away. The clouds have severed my attachment to him, removing my heart and placing it far away from him. The clouds do not like to have fun. They will not allow me to enjoy myself.

At first, Patrick is perplexed, unable to understand what suddenly went so wrong. I know he wonders if it is something he said. No doubt he blames himself. No doubt he interprets my sudden change as a result of something he said or did, or a change in my feelings towards him. The band plays "Little

Red Corvette" and the lights are turned low while all the students dance. Everyone that is, except for me. And Patrick who now thinks he's a fool for bringing this dud of a date.

I ask him to take me home early. We say little as I bid him goodnight and leave him standing alone on the front porch.

September 15, 1984
Wt: 99 lbs.

My parents want to talk to me alone. My mother does not try to mask her worry, it is written in the faint beginnings of lines across her forehead, traces that were not there five months ago. On the other hand, my father's disguise is uneven, as he looks worried one minute, and in the next resumes his good-natured smile. I try to disguise my discomfort.

They have not said much about my weight since I've been home. My mother has fought the urge to ask me to please eat, to be more conscious of eating healthy. I know that we are now seated together at this kitchen table upon their request to discuss my eating habits. No matter how carefully I've tried to hide my diet, there's no way to escape the peering eyes and silent inquiries of those who live under the same roof.

They have tried repeatedly to get me to join them in family dinners. They refuse to give up. Night after night they ask. But I always refuse, feigning any one of a multitude of excuses of either being too busy or needing to run before it gets dark outside. They have tried to be patient. No longer do they encourage my running. It is no longer the same enthusiastic symbol of achievement as it was at the beginning of the summer. They realize that the running, like the food aversion, has turned tail and transformed before their very eyes into another monster, another inexplicable force that controls me in such an unhealthy manner. They no longer compliment me on my weight loss. Now their looks are stern, looks that say it all, looks that demand, looks that plead. Invisible thought bubbles that float over their heads are filled with all the things they wish they could say but do not. I am met with looks of shock, glances of helplessness as they watch me wash and tear lettuce pieces, toss them on a plate, and pretend to enjoy this meal as much as if it were prime rib.

My mother speaks of her friend whose daughter will not eat either. She says it is a sickness called anorexia. Says the daughter has struggled with it for three years. Says the daughter is the same age as me. Says the daughter is so weak now that all she can do is lie on the couch. Says her friend and her friend's husband haven't been able to do anything to help her gain back the weight. Says the girl now weighs eighty pounds.

Eighty pounds, I think to myself, feeling how much greater her accomplishments are over that of mine. *If only I could lose that much weight and get down to her size.* I feel inadequate compared to such an accomplished girl.

My mother's voice trembles as she once again relays this story. I've already heard it a dozen times. It is as if somehow my mother views this as motivation for me to change my habits. Yet I remain unmoved and unmotivated to change, even after hearing it over and over. I do not personally know the girl to whom she refers, but I feel I understand her. Without knowing her, I know that this girl will not willingly put on a single pound any more than I am willing to do so. No one can force her to eat, not even herself.

My mother's voice trembles and I feel guilty. I do not want my mother to worry about me. I don't want to cause her pain. I wish she would just forget about me, focus on someone else, leave me alone, quit judging me. I want to be left alone with my diet and my running and the gray clouds in my mind that will not go away, for these are the only things that I feel do belong to me. No one can help. I don't want help. Their help I don't want because there could only be a single outcome – that I will gain back the weight, that I will be fat again. Any help will only serve to revert back into that girl I despise so much. Why do they want me to be fat?

My father has taken off work to be present. Their expressions are somber, and I know they mean business. I know they want to say all the things they have not said before. I will hear it all now. It is written all over their faces. I cannot escape. I fear what they have to say.

The kitchen table is dented and scratched. I pretend to be interested in my great-grandmother's pie safe that leans against the wall, an austere dark mahogany antique that my mother re-finished herself. Wallpaper sketched with chickens and hens attempts to perk up the somber mood.

"Daddy and I are worried about you," my mother begins. She wears an old pair of blue jeans and one of my brother's shirts. Her frosted hair is curled and her lips bear a fresh swipe of Passion Pink.

My father nods in agreement. His manicured hands rest on the table. His fingers sift one against another, indicative of his nervousness. I wish I weren't sitting here with them. I do not want to hear anything they have to say.

As I look into my father's face, it is the first time that I have ever seen him appear helpless. My dad, the strong one, the supporter. He is at a loss, and it is my fault. Guilt. Guilt. Guilt. My mother seems to instinctively know how at a loss for words my father is at the moment.

Speaking as gently as possible, she says, "We just want to help you."

"I don't need help," I insist.

She listens, nods and continues. "We've been biting our tongues for months now. We haven't said much to you about your eating habits. We thought at first this was just an extension of your earlier diet. Now we realize it's gone far, far past that. This is no longer a mere diet, and it hasn't been for a very long time."

"I don't want to get fat," is the only thing I can think of to say, and the beginnings of anger begin to stir inside.

"You're not fat," she insists, her voice raised just enough to get her point across. She wants to scream but my mother never screams. She never yells. She never hollers. She never cusses. She knows how to get any point across by maintaining a calm demeanor.

"You are not fat. Have you looked at yourself in the mirror? You're skin and bones...skin and bones."

My dad interrupts. "I can see the bones in your neck, in your shoulders. Sticking out like those starving people in National Geographic." He winces and turns away.

I feel exposed, too exposed, and wish I had a sweater in which to hide in, to cover up my arms, to button high at the neck. Anything to feel less exposed. Anything in which to hide and disappear.

My mother continues. "The not eating, the running...you're not eating properly. I don't think you even eat five-hundred calories a day."

More like three-hundred, I think to myself although I say nothing, clinging tightly to my secret in order to avoid further exposure. It begins to dawn on me that my mother, who has never counted a calorie in her life, has suddenly acquired this knowledge. She has been learning, teaching herself, wasting time she does not have.

"I'm healthier than I've ever been," I state without much conviction.

"That's not true and you know it." Then she pauses, and re-considers this last statement. "But then again, maybe you don't know it. I believe you really do see yourself as fat, that you sincerely believe you are healthy. I believe you really don't see yourself as you are, how you look, how thin you've become. I believe when you look in the mirror you see something else, something the rest of us can't see. I really believe that you don't see it, that you don't realize what you are doing to your body, to your heart."

My anger begins to inwardly boil at this invasion of privacy. She knows nothing. She will never understand. How can

I expect her to understand when I don't even understand, when I cannot even begin to explain it. There's no point in even trying.

"How do you know so much about my body?" I quip.

"Your daddy and I have been doing some research," she says, ignoring my smart-alecky tone. "There's a rising population of young women just like you who all of a sudden stop eating. They start out just as you did, by going on a diet. But then it escalates into something much worse, and no one seems to be able to explain why. These girls, they keep losing weight, exercising all the time. Getting thinner and thinner until they reach the point of emaciation. Just like you."

"Emaciated?" I say. Of course I know I am far from emaciation. In the mirror, I do not see a thin girl, only the flab on my thighs that refuses to slim down even after all the running. I see the fleshed-out cheeks of baby fat on my face that won't budge no matter how few calories I consume. Even my stomach feels bloated. *Emaciated* would pertain to me if I were forty pounds lighter. It is most definitely not a term that pertains to me.

My mother is not finished. "These girls think they're fat when they're not. It's a sickness, something new, something that doctors are just beginning to deal with and try to understand and treat. What they do know is that it occurs mainly in young women your age."

I don't know how to respond. Yes, I've heard the term, heard about my mother's friend's daughter who supposedly has 'this disease'. Can't everyone just leave me alone? Can't they see that I just need to lose a little bit more weight and then everything will be fine? "Your daddy and I have talked with a doctor. He's located here in town and is a renowned expert in this field. He treats women with this disease. Women with eating disorders. We want you to go talk to him."

I remain glued to my chair, unable to budge. *Warning! Warning! Warning!* Internal warning signals begin to flash. *Possible exposure risk should I talk to anyone.* I don't want to change a thing. I don't want to lose what I've worked so hard to attain. I don't want any help because their kind of help will only make me fat. There is no way I can begin to explain all that goes through my mind. No one would understand. They would all laugh. They would think me ridiculous. I have no intention of speaking with any so-called expert about this. What does he know about me anyway? There is nothing to discuss.

"Why?" I ask.

"To see if he can help you," she replies.

"I don't need help," I insist. And yet everything inside tells me that I definitely need help. I need to turn my life around without reverting back to the darkness of yesterday. I need to know where to go from here. I need for the sadness to go away. I don't even know why it is there. But I know there is no one who will understand, no one who can help.

There once was a time, years ago, when I desperately needed help. But no one came to my rescue. Why would it be any different now? Perhaps I am meant to solve my own problems. I don't want to burden anyone. I don't want them to see my problems, my fears, my worries, and judge me as pathetic. I couldn't stand it. Better to keep this contained mess to myself.

And then I can see her mind moving, the revelation as she begins to fully realize the magnitude of this wall, the impenetrable fortress that refuses any help. She realizes there is nothing more she can say to move me or change my mind. And at that moment I hate myself more than I have ever hated myself before. I hate myself for putting them in this position, for causing them to feel so helpless, for all the worry I've created, and for being so adamant in my refusal of their help. With all their might they are trying to reach out to me, trying to offer any olive branch or flotation device they can think of. But I cannot take it. I cannot take it. And this continues to cause even greater pain.

"Then," she says quietly, "if you don't need help for yourself, would you please go for us, for me and Daddy?"

My father glances up at me, trying to maintain his usual upbeat composure, his cheery attempt to hold together the broken pieces of this family. But, before my very eyes, I watch as it suddenly washes away in helpless defeat, a silent surrender before the raising of the white flag.

"Please," he whispers. "Please do it for us."

September 16, 1984
Wt: 99 lbs.

I do not want to be a laughingstock when I visit the doctor. I do not want to enter his office and have him take one look at me, this big 'ol cow of a girl, and say out loud for all to hear, "*What are you doing in my office? I only treat girls with eating disorders. You obviously have no eating disorder because you are too fat. You must have made some mistake.*" I imagine this declaration to be followed by the howling laughter of both him and his staff at the joke my parents have played on all of us. I need to lose more weight before I meet him.

September 18, 1984
Wt: 96 lbs.

I go alone, entering the black-glass façade of a four-story building in the heart of mid-town, home to the most expensive commercial real estate in the city. The lobby is graced with limestone floors, marbled walls and brass elevators. Taking in the lavish interior, I know this appointment will cost my parents a fortune. I know they don't have the money for this, not when there will be three of us in college this fall. Guilt. Guilt. Guilt.

I take the elevator to the third floor and search for his suite. The narrow hallway is quiet and cool like a mausoleum. Burgundy carpet pads the floor. I give the receptionist my name and take a seat in the empty waiting room. It is so quiet in here, and so chilly. I wish I'd remembered to bring a sweater. I am always so cold, even in the middle of this scorching summer. Always cold.

Within a minute, an inner door opens and I am greeted by a tall middle-aged man wearing a pink shirt and yellow tie. He possesses a kindly countenance as he smiles, warmly extends a hand and introduces himself. He shows me into his office where outdoor sunlight is shielded by a long wall of vertical blinds. A dozen framed diplomas flank one wall, each mounted in wood. In front of his desk, two leather wingbacks face each other as if engaged in an inanimate conversation.

He gestures towards the empty seats, leaving the decision for me to choose. Then he takes a seat in a velvet wingback behind his desk.

"I want to thank you for coming in," he begins. "I know you didn't want to but I'm glad that you did." His voice is gentle and sincere.

I nod. *Correct,* I think to myself, *I did not want to come.* "I'm only here because I promised my parents," I say.

He nods as if he's already heard the identical response on numerous occasions. He gets straight to the point. "You don't think you have a problem, do you?"

"No sir. I don't."

"Okay then. Let's not even talk about eating."

Relief. I can't believe my ears as this isn't at all what I expected.

He continues. "Are you able to tell me what's been going on inside your head?"

I stare at him, stare into the whites of his eyes magnified behind a pair of silver-rimmed bifocals. I recognize the same expression as that of my mother when we lunched at the cafeteria, the moment when she looked at my eyes during that single moment in time and saw the briefest glimmer of the true distress. His eyes possess the same gentleness of trying to understand, of being open to what it is I have to say, of knowing something is wrong. He poses the question in such a manner that suggests there is a true problem, one that has nothing to do with my weight. One that has nothing to do with food.

Unlike the opportunities to speak before, I want to explain, to tell him about the washing machine set permanently on spin cycle, the gray clouds that won't go away, the sadness that never leaves. I want to explain but I cannot find the words. I am unable to place a finger on any one particular thing for it is all coiled into one cumbersome jumbled mess that I can't begin to untangle. One tangled mess that I can't unravel. One neatly packaged box filled with too many emotions for one person to carry. I have been afraid to even try opening this box or unraveling all the knots for fear that one loose brick will suddenly force the entire house to collapse in a heap of debris and rubble. I wouldn't know how to deal with, how to fix what's broken let alone even know where to begin. And it would no doubt result in a single ending: my getting fat, reverting back into that lost girl I despise.

I want to explain but I don't know where to begin. I don't know what it is that spins and spews in my head, only that it hurts and is heavy and that I want it to go away. Suddenly, I feel overwhelmed. I glance down into my lap, into the vivid canary cotton of my embroidered Mexican dress, a festive exterior that belies the drab, gray, truer interior of my soul.

Tears begin to well, adding to my frustration. Droplets begin to ease down my face and into my lap, forming a pool of moisture.

He remains seated silently as he reaches for a tissue and hands it to me. My shoulders start to shake as I break into sobs. The sadness is coming. It is big. A huge sadness that builds daily, a diligent force with no rhyme or reason other than to ensure its presence is not forgotten. The sadness is coming and it won't turn away. It refuses to hide any longer. The sadness is coming, tremors felt along the ocean floor, reverberating throughout undiscovered sea caverns filled with swimming creatures that have never seen the sun and sunken pirate ships filled with gold. I feel it breaking free, loosening its bonds through the dominant power of sheer will, and I can no longer hold it back. The wall is cracking.

I continue sobbing, embarrassed at how ridiculous I must appear, but at the same time unable to hold back the physical release of all the anguish. I am embarrassed that I cannot stop crying. Here I sit in a fancy psychiatrist's office, wasting my parents' hard-earned money by bawling like an idiot.

"Jackie..." There is tenderness in his voice. I do not look up but I feel him lean slightly towards me as he lowers his voice and simply asks, "Why are you so sad?"

Upon hearing this, the sobs intensify. I try to wipe my eyes but the tissue is wet as a dishrag. As is the next tissue and the next until perhaps a half hour passes before I am able to somewhat calm down and regain some semblance of composure. My face is swollen, hot and red. I finally meet his eyes, he who stares at me with such earnest. His fingers are laced together in front of his face.

"I miss Julian," are the only words that escape my lips, an unexpected declaration that had not been in my mind just a minute ago. It is the first thing that comes to mind, and the instant I utter this truth, I realize there are so many things I miss.

"Julian," he says as if hearing the name for the very first time. He says it again. "Julian." Only this time he says it with deep emotion, clearly enunciating every syllable because he has instantly grasped the fact that there is deep hidden meaning attached to this name. He says it in a way that shows he understands just how much is attached to this person, five letters that represent *something, something real and important.*

"Julian," he repeats. "You loved Julian very much, didn't you?"

He grasps this instantly, quicker than anyone else has for that matter. He has grasped the source of my pain, and for me that is enough.

I nod to reply. Yes, I loved him very much. I loved him so much and now that he is not here I am lost. I am always lost.

"I can see how much he meant to you," he says.

It is the affirmation that I need to hear although I do not know why. To be seen, for someone to understand. I am grateful for his ability to pick up on this so quickly. He understands. At last, somebody understands. It is a relief. And a release. I begin to wonder why he is able to pick up on this so quickly when others could not.

He ventures further. "Jackie, is this the first time you've faced rejection?"

I stare at him blankly as if this term, rejection, is the farthest thing from my mind. Rejection. How does he know this? How could he possibly know this about me? I do not ever want anybody to view me this way – rejected, scorned, cast off.

When I fail to respond, he continues. "Is there something that occurred before, perhaps a long time ago, when you were also faced with the pain of rejection?" He stares at me with that look that sees straight into my insides, that part of me that I do not want anyone to see. How does he know this? How does he know? Have my parents told him anything about my past? Not much delving into the past is required for me to realize he has quickly found the crux of so much pain. Still, how does he know?

Rejection. The memories of the eight long tortuous years of grade school return to my unwilling mind as I try to push them right back into the secret recesses where they have dwelled in dormancy all these years. I do not want to be reminded. I do not want to re-live those years. I would rather be dead than re-live those years.

I know this doctor has latched onto something big, something that could explain a lot. Something that could explain everything. Or at least most of everything. Yet it is not something I ever care to re-visit. I cannot discuss it. Not now. Not ever. Perhaps it would help. I wonder. But I dare not venture back in time to those earlier years. I cannot sink any further than I already have.

I stare at him stone-faced and say, "'I cannot talk about that."

He nods his head, not wanting to push. "Okay."

Then, with sudden about-face, I ask, "Do you think I have an eating disorder?"

He places his large hands firmly on the cherry desk top and demands my gaze. "Yes I do."

"Why?" I ask.

"I can tell just by looking at you. Even though that oversized dress has no shape, I see that you are perhaps thirty pounds underweight. My guess is somewhere between ninety-eight and one-hundred-one pounds. Your calf muscles are also developed, indicating to me that you run long-distance. And my guess is also that your exercise exceeds more than your daily caloric intake. To lose the amount of weight you have requires an intake of no more than 400 calories per day. That, and the running which you obviously do. To do all of this, Jackie, takes an inordinate amount of discipline, a will of steel to control the dieting and the hunger you no doubt feel at all times. And, my dear, you have learned to master your willpower. You've learned how to control every aspect of your weight, right down to the last ounce."

I sit back and stare at him, astonished. I have to admit I am impressed with his knowledge, how he seems to know so much about me, how he has guessed my weight correctly, how he understands the inner battle that controls the hunger and the calories. I am impressed and even a little intrigued because I assumed that *I* was the only one in the world privy to my private thoughts and habits.

He continues. "Very little is known about this disease. It seemed to unearth itself only recently, like an underground volcano that suddenly erupted without warning. Therefore, there is much we still don't understand, and much we still must learn if we are to help the growing number of young women afflicted with anorexia."

I think to myself, *there is no way you'll ever understand. There is no doctor or psychiatrist or anyone in the entire medical profession who will ever understand because they cannot physically see what's going on inside my head. It will never make sense because they cannot look inside. They cannot see the gray clouds or feel the burden of their weight. They cannot see a mind in constant overdrive, fatigued by the overwhelming fears and anxieties. They will never imagine how large and consuming these things are. They do not see that all of these things have overtaken me and now control me. I am their prisoner and I want out, but there is no way out.*

He adds, "What we do know is this: 98% of the cases are female, approximately between the ages of 16 and 24 although we are now seeing cases involving much younger girls as well as women in their twenties and thirties. Generally, though, they are from middle to upper-income families. A high percentage would be perceived as perfectionists. They have high expectations of themselves and of others; they are internally motivated."

He mentions a few other facts, but I am no longer listening. I am focused on something else he said earlier, when he referred to it as a disease.

"How can you call it a disease?" I question. "Cancer is a disease. Multiple sclerosis is a disease. Leukemia is a disease. I don't know, it just seems so...so insulting to those with real diseases." I know in my heart I have caused this whereas others do not cause their cancer or other diseases.

He nods, taking my point seriously. "It's a disease of the mind," he replies. "It starts out innocently enough, as a diet. Nine times out of ten these girls merely set out to lose some weight, to shed a few pounds. But then it escalates.

The weight is lost, usually rapidly, but the girl looks in the mirror and cannot see the slimmed-down version standing before her. In fact, in her mind, she sees herself as bigger, fatter, and worse-off than before. Even though at this point the girl weighs far less than what she medically should. She does not see herself as thin. Instead she sees something in the mirror that the rest of us cannot see."

He continues. "The intricacies of the mind are still relatively unknown. However, we do know one thing for a fact, and it is this – your mind will believe what you tell it to believe. It does not have the automatic capacity to instinctively determine right from wrong. These differences – right, wrong, sad, happy, mad – are all things that we program into our minds. If you tell yourself over and over that you are too fat, that you will be as big as an elephant if you consume an extra hundred calories, then your mind will eventually believe it. Even though this may be a false reality. The mind is loyal to its owner and will faithfully obey what it is taught. And once that happens, once the mind believes things that are not true, the cycle of danger and destruction begins, a cycle that is very difficult to unravel."

I listen to his words carefully. They make sense but still I do not wholly believe they pertain to me. I *am* fat. Surely he can see it, surely he is just being polite to my face.

He looks at me, waiting for a reaction. I offer none. "Can we discuss your health?" he asks.

I'm tired and not in the mood to listen to much more. I'm tired and all I want to do is to go home and go back to sleep. I feel I could sleep through the rest of the day, into the night until tomorrow.

Recognizing that I'm spent, he realizes he has a short window to say what he has to say. "You're in a situation, Jackie, that is not going to stop. It will only worsen and you will begin to further weaken. This will not stop, not until you get some professional help. I can help you. I've helped other girls like you."

"I don't need any help," I say.

"That's another symptom of this disease. All the girls say that they don't need professional help. They profess this aloud but inside they know it isn't true. Indeed they do want help but there are too many doubts about whether a medical professional could truly help. The thought I want to leave you with today is the eventual toll that not eating will have on your body."

"But I'm in perfect health," I argue. "I eat healthy foods." *Apples, lettuce, tomatoes, mustard & water sweetened with low-calorie sweetener.* "I run three miles a day. I'd call that perfect health." Half of my mind actually believes this. The other half, the side that struggles against reform, wants to invalidate this statement.

"It may seem like that on the outside," he counters, "to others who view you in the same manner as one would admire a rare china tureen in an antique shop. In our society, it is deemed admirable to be thin. By others who view thinness as the perfect ideal, the ultimate status symbol that suggests one has everything under control, that one has the world by the tail, so to speak."

"But nothing is in control, other than your control over food." He pauses for a second, then backs up and says, "You said you didn't want to discuss weight so we won't. This isn't about food. Right now, you're in a critical situation, critical of it escalating even further, of damaging your body worse than you already have."

"Damaging my body?!" I stammer. In my mind, my body is invincible. I never see it getting too old or permanently sick or failing me. Those things happen to other people, not to me. I am young even though too often I feel aged beyond my years.

He says, "Long-term lack of proper nutrition takes a heavy toll on health: heart palpitations, mineral loss, bone density loss, dizziness, liver damage, kidney damage. The list goes on and on and on."

While he continues through the long list of health consequences, my mind does not entertain any of it seriously. It is as if I hear, '*blah blah blah blah blah blah blah blah blah blah,*' for I feel as if my body will eternally be seventeen years old.

He continues to drone on. "Many girls have died from this, literally died from malnutrition and heart attacks by the stresses placed on vital organs from years of food deprivation."

What do I care about any of this? I am only twenty. Other people die. Not me. My body is invincible; it will never fail me. It runs as far as I command it to. It survives on the few calories I allow. It has even survived the traumas of the past. It is obvious that he is referring to someone else, other girls. What does he know about me? Nothing. Therefore, how could he help? He cannot.

"I would like for you to enter a treatment center," he says.

Now I'm ready to get up and leave. I uncross my legs and begin to stand, but he gestures me back down. "There's one here in town. I know what you're thinking: a hospital. But it's not like that. Not at all. It's a comfortable setting. Other girls are there. The treatment focuses on helping you to overcome your addiction."

"I don't have an addiction," I lie. He just wants to take away my control. He wants me to be helpless. I've been in helpless situations before and would therefore never intentionally place myself in such a spot again.

"I want you to go, and your parents want you to go too," he says.

"You've discussed this with my parents?" I ask.

He nods. "Yes. They didn't want to bring it up for fear of making everything even worse, for fear of scaring you into eating even less. They're terrified. They just want you to get better, and they don't know how to do it other than for you to enter a treatment facility."

Guilt Guilt Guilt. My parents are terrified. Even still, I know I will not go. I'll never go to a treatment center where people I don't know pry and probe into my past, where other girls walk the halls and judge every aspect of my exterior and my personality. I will not go and be exposed in this manner. They cannot help me. I cannot even help myself. I cannot allow anything to unravel, not when I have worked so hard to control it so perfectly, rolled up in a tight little ball even though I know the harm this has caused. No no no.

"I'll think about it," I lie again.

Then, I stand and exit the door without saying thank you or goodbye. I take the elevator back down to the lobby and exit the building into the humid air that is difficult to breathe. I walk into the bright afternoon sunshine whose yellow rays of life I do not see due to the barrier of the gray clouds that continue to weigh heavily on my mind. I will never return.

September 25, 1984
Wt: 99 lbs.

The ridicule was there for eight long years, an eternity to a little girl who wanted nothing more than to be accepted.

The ridicule builds up over time, creating an invisible fortress brick by brick, stone by stone, layer by layer. Until one day the fortress becomes a home in which the little girl lives. She has two choices: either to remain hidden within the fortress where she keeps to herself and minds her own business and keeps her mind occupied so that the loneliness does not overwhelm her. Or, she can open the doors of the fortress and venture out.

Should she choose the second alternative, the fortress shall then swing open its mighty door and the little girl will stand in its threshold just long enough to get a whiff of the foulness of the ridicule that awaits her should she take one step beyond.

Because no reward lies in choosing the second alternative, the mighty fortress door remains tightly shut. The girl therefore dwells within the fortress that becomes her second home, an imaginary structure in which to escape when she is not under her parents' roof. She dwells within the chilly confines of the fortress, and over time begins to believe that she deserves to live here, that she deserves to be alone, that she does not deserve friends, that she is wholly worthy of being a laughingstock to be incessantly mocked and ridiculed. Tempting it is to leave her capsule for fear that time moves forward without her. Isolation and loneliness become overpowering to the point where she feels she cannot breathe. There is no one to talk to. No one would understand.

Years of living in the fortress help to preserve her sanity. But the mocking calls and jeers and stabs and words of ridicule have somehow still managed to penetrate through the slight cracks in the window frames, through the tiny holes of mortar. Over a long period of time, after hearing the negativity repeated over and over and over and over, the little girl, consciously and unconsciously, begins to believe what she hears. She believes the negative words that others say about her. *It must be true,* she tells herself. *It must be true. For why else would they say these things? I am but one person while they form a midst of many, and surely the forces of truth summoned by this court of many negates what it is I feel inside.*

At first, the girl does not believe the cruel words of the Mean Girls. However, over time they eventually become a part of her. She assumes a new identity, one that she was not born with and never knew before she arrived at this school. She assumes an invisible coat of gray, handed to her by the Mean Girls. It threads are weathered and torn, and moths have chewed away at its wool. It is the cloak nobody else wants or wears, except for her.

It took some getting used to. The gray cloak was not fully worn that first day when it was handed to the little girl.

At first she slips in a single arm into one of the sleeves, and she wears it like that, half-worn while the other half hangs at her side. Over time she gets used to wearing the single sleeve until finally one day she places the uncovered arm inside the unused sleeve. Now the coat hangs fully on her frame. The Mean Girls think it suits her well.

The gray coat has a musty odor. The girl becomes used to wearing it day in and day out but she does not like it. She does not like its gray color or its musty smell. It is not a pretty coat; it is not bright and cheery like the ones the other girls wear. This coat makes her feel ugly. She does not like to wear it and longs for a coat like the other girls, one with vivid bold colors, one without holes, one that bears the fresh new scent of a fine department store.

She longs to wear a different coat, but this is that which was handed to her by the judgment of her peers. She wears the coat and continues to wish that she was not cast in this macabre play with the role of The Girl in the Gray Coat. She longs for the day when she will no longer wear it, but she knows that day is far away, light years away in a future that she can neither see nor imagine.

She wears the coat always. With a single exception.

The coat is shed when comfort is sought behind the keys of her piano. During these brief respites, the coat is cast aside as she plays the melancholic night music of Chopin and the sonatas of Beethoven and Mozart. No one can touch her as long as her fingers are attached to the ivories, when she enters and commands her private realm of music. It is a realm in which she brings back to life the manuscript pages of notes and key changes written by classical composers dead now for centuries.

The music of the dead springs back to life through her fingertips, but it is not death that the little girl feels. Rather, it is a life-giving force that provides the sole source of nutrition to her soul. It fuels her body and breathes new air back into her fractured heart and injured mindset. It assures her that *this* can never be taken away from her, that *this* is hers and hers alone.

The rhapsodies of the dead assemble into a full orchestra within her mind and play that which only her ears can hear. The music is their gift to her, and she pours what enters through her imagination as inaudible sound waves onto the keys of the piano. This symphony of musicians welcomes her back again and again, and places her at the helm of the stage underneath a single spotlight that shines throughout the duration of her solo concerts. The sounds of the dead welcome her with open arms no matter how frequently she returns. They never disappoint. They never judge. They only embrace.

Those who dwell outside of the fortress and wear the vivid coats of the living are not aware of the girl's attachment to music. The girl will never tell them about it. She will never reveal the one outside source that gives her life, that temporarily restores her to wholeness. She will not risk what the others might do or say should they discover her private realm of music. She will not risk the certainty that they would find fault with that which is most sacred to her. No doubt it would be scrutinized mercilessly, shred to pieces, kicked at like an old tire, and then carelessly discarded in a heap of wreckage. No, the girl will not betray her loyal source.

October 3, 1984
Wt: 99 lbs.

Met two new friends in the university chorale.

This class is the simplest of courses where the single requirement is that one show up on time and sing. I expected the class to be easy. What I didn't expect was to discover two new buddies and to have this much fun. The common bond is music, one that is instantly formed as we begin to discover identical taste in movies. Helene says her favorites are The Sound of Music and The Wizard of Oz. Margaret says these are her favorites as well. I agree.

Today marks the instructor's birthday. Her elaborate musical resume includes major roles with the city opera as well as The Broadway Series. The theatre is her real home, and therefore she offers much through her experience. Helene instigates a surprise in which the entire class sings 'Happy Birthday'. But this is no ordinary song, in fact quite unlike the singsong version of children settled around a cherry cake lit with burning candles. This version consists of two dozen singers, male and female, who convert a simple melody into an improvised twelve-part harmony masterpiece. Baritone, bass, tenor, alto, soprano, second-soprano ... all unite in separate streams that meet at the mouth of the river. Each unrehearsed line combines with another to join into one beautiful, broad, bold opera.

The teacher seemed impressed even though she is used to the big stage.

The song stays with me throughout the remainder of the day.

October 5, 1984
Wt: 99 lbs.

My mother says she's happy I have made new friends. She's especially happy that they are female because she says there's nothing like your girlfriends who are there for you when you need them. She says you'll count on them, and in return they'll count on you for the rest of your life.

October 8, 1984
Wt: 100 lbs.

I return home late after an evening out with my new friends. I laughed all night. I am starting to feel like my old self again as the laughter slowly returns. I have not laughed like this in a long time.

I arrive home happy and tired. It is nearly one a.m. My parents are sleeping at the other end of the house. Richard and Leslie are away at school. My other two siblings are asleep in their rooms. I have no curfew now that I am twenty. I come and go as I please and my father no longer waits up for me like he did when I was in high school.

I am tired. I need sleep. But I am hungry, much too hungry to fall instantly into slumber. This hunger will keep me awake as long as it remains unheeded. But I know that I cannot eat anything. I can't risk the chance of gaining back any of the weight. I cannot get fat. I won't get fat. Not after all this dieting and exercise. I won't lose my willpower no matter how hungry I feel at the moment. I peek into the refrigerator and consider making a salad.

Instead, I decide to bake brownies, knowing full well that it will take an hour before they are finished. I am too tired to stay awake another hour but I decide to do so anyway. I will make brownies for my family.

I find a box of Betty Crocker in the pantry. There are plenty of eggs in the refrigerator. I pour chocolate mix into a bowl, then add the oil, water and eggs, and begin to stir and stir. I stir the thick batter of chocolate that further intoxicates with its rich cocoa aroma. I taste a tiny spoonful that immediately awakens my taste buds and begs for more. The chocolate tastes so good, the rarest of treats in a weak moment of collapsed strength. Its sweetness nourishes and demands another taste. I dip the spoon back into the batter and taste another bite. This one tastes even better than the first. The hunger is now fully awakened, not satisfied in the least. It demands for *more, more, more.*

I envision myself taking yet another bite, then another, and then another until the bowl is empty before it even gets poured into the baking dish. I am that hungry. But I will not lose my control. Two bites are enough. Already these two bites have necessitated the need to run an extra mile tomorrow. Perhaps two miles.

The oven bell dings to indicate the set temperature is reached. I pour the batter into a pan, place it in the oven and then set the timer for forty-five minutes. I am so tired now that I could go straight to bed without removing makeup or clothes.

I sit in the den rocking chair and turn on the television. Impatiently checking my watch, I realize there is a long wait ahead, a wait that seems that much longer because of my fatigue. Fatty jumps into my lap, curls in a ball and falls instantly asleep. I pet his old soft fur and he continues to purr despite the obvious vivid images within his kitty dreams. My eyes strain to focus on a late-night movie. But the urge to sleep begs for mercy, to give in to it, for once to surrender to the primal hunger.

I am awakened by the second ring of the oven timer. The brownies are done. The rich chocolate smells heavenly and the aroma fills the sleeping house. I worry that it will awaken my parents.

I set the glass dish on a potholder, turn off the lights and go to bed. Somebody will enjoy this dessert tomorrow. It just won't be me.

October 10, 1984
Wt: 101 lbs.

Casual glances turn into anger as my mother pleads with me not to bake any more brownies in the wee hours of the morning.

"You bake for us all the time but you never eat what you bake," she says. "You never eat the chocolate chip cookies or the fudge bars or the brownies that you bake alone in the kitchen, at night while the rest of us sleep. Please do not do this anymore."

October 12, 1984
Wt: 101 lbs.

I long for days past when I could eat a steak and baked potato and not worry about whether or not it will make me gain weight. I dream of eating a hamburger and onion rings and not feeling like I need to run ten miles to override the calories.

It seems a lifetime ago when I did not feel the need to eat in secrecy. I keep it to myself, and never tell a soul about my secret treks to Hamburgers by Charlie where I order the biggest jalapeno burger on the menu, plus onion rings, then sit in my car, alone and in secret. I do not tell a soul how I pick apart the burger, slowly shredding the buns into tiny pieces before discarding them into the paper sack, the whole while thinking about the damaging repercussions of all those fattening carbohydrates. I dare not mention the fact that I nibble around the edges of the meat patty, savoring the flavors of grease and charcoal. I keep to myself the fact that I eat perhaps an eighth of the meat before quickly relinquishing the remainder of that as well to the paper bag for fear that I will lose all control of my will and eat it in its entirety. I dare not mention that the only parts of the burger that are fully consumed are the tomatoes, pickles and lettuce that bear the drippings of ketchup and mayonnaise and mustard, condiments that somehow seem like forbidden desserts.

I pick apart that hamburger in the same manner that the Mean Girls once picked me apart.

I do not tell anyone of this habit. I am ashamed of it. I am so ashamed of this. I am so ashamed that the hunger keeps drawing me back, again and again, to the same burger joint where the same process is repeated over and over. I am ashamed that I am such a freak.

October 13, 1984
Wt: 103 lbs

Teddy phones to relay some good news: I was nominated for Homecoming Court.

"*Huh?*" is the only answer I can muster from a brain in shock. I am stunned, and immediately assume there has been a mistake. I think he is joking as he usually is.

No, he says, he's not kidding.

Enthusiasm peppers his speech as he begins to explain. He hurries through a long list of details, and ends by telling me the event will take place in two weeks. He tells me to go buy a dress and find a date.

We hang up and I remain standing there, stunned. In my mind, I rationalize that I haven't made enough friends at my new school to warrant this honor. I continue to wonder if this is some kind of joke. Surely he is joking. These types of honors are reserved for others, for my prettier sisters, the ones who are popular and are cheerleaders. These milestones are always reserved for others, never for me. But Teddy was serious and this is for real.

Who will I take? While I have many male friends at school, there are no romantic interests. Could I ask one of them? Would they mind my asking them? Would they even go or would they consider it a joke? Would they mind wearing the required coat and tie or enduring the embarrassment of escorting me?

What will I wear? Nothing in my closet will do. I do not own a proper dress. I must buy a new dress, one that doesn't make me look fat. And I have but two short weeks to find one. Somewhere in between all of that there are also three scheduled exams that need my full concentration. Where will I find the time?

My mother is thrilled and seems as though she's not the least bit surprised. *See? I told you,* she says. *You're making more progress than you think.*

What I can't figure out is how I got nominated when I feel so lonely inside, so isolated. Can't everyone see the gray clouds that hover above my head? Can they see the clouds that weigh me down every day? Inside I feel one way, but they must see something else, a vision I do not realize.

Two weeks. Two short weeks. Who will be my escort? Will I have to stand in front of everyone to be viewed by all?

Yes.

Will I be judged? Will they judge how I look? Two short weeks. Wait until my sisters hear about this. What will they think? How will they react? Will they be happy? Of course they will. They'll probably be just as surprised as I am.

As the questions begin to flow, a sense of dread begins to overwhelm me. It fills my stomach with heaviness, with fears of competition, fears of failure, failure in front of the entire student body. Fears of being exposed, having all my bad traits revealed and then judged, the outcome of which I assume will always be negative.

I am not good enough, not pretty enough, not thin enough, not smart enough, not worthy enough. I have a lot of work to do in order to prepare for this. A few more pounds to shed. A dress to buy. A date to find. I need to work on my hair. I can't stand up there in front of everybody and make a fool out of myself. Who can I ask that won't turn me down?

Anxiety. I feel it setting in already. I don't know how I'll manage to sleep for the next two weeks. Panic begins to set in. How will I do this? How will I stand in front of everybody waiting for that final judgment call of whether I will be a winner or a loser?

I want the anxiety and panic to go away. I don't know how to deal with this. I can't figure out how to deal with this. This time it's too large to run it away with the many miles jogged along the pavement. I just want it to go away. I want the gray to disappear. I want to disappear.

October 17, 1984
Wt: 102 lbs.

Opting for the course of safety, I ask an escort who I know is safe, who I know without a doubt will not reject me. He never has rejected me before and I know he never will. My father.

After all, it is his alma-mater, where he was a cheerleader twenty-five years earlier. His happiness at having been asked touches me, and makes me feel that much surer in my decision. He's been whistling happily ever since.

October 25, 1984
Wt: 101 lbs.

Dad bought a white orchid and pinned it to my dress, a clingy navy knit with a high neck, long sleeves and cut just above the knee.

As my name is called, my father walks me to center stage. I should have been terrified but instead felt strangely calm for I had my father's arm to hold, and I felt that no matter who won, everything was going to be all right.

When the Grand Marshall announces Deborah's name as the winner, I am not surprised. She deserves it, and she looks beautiful too.

Dad wanted to stay for the dance. I could have easily gone home at that point, but I didn't want to disappoint him. My father makes friends easily. He saw many of his old friends – those who attended the university with him and whose children now attend school with me. Others he knows from his business or through his many social networks.

My dad knows no stranger and easily maneuvers a room, meeting new people as easily as he drinks a glass of water. He introduces himself to not only every girl on the court but to their dates as well. My outgoing social father is completely in his element here, and I wish I were more like him. I wish I had his happy nature, his complete lack of fear around others, his outgoing manner that enables him to walk into a room where he knows no one and within ten minutes is able to not only name each individual but also deliver an oral recitation of their background.

My father makes the evening easy for me. He understands how prohibitive my shy nature can be and therefore goes out of his way to introduce me to as many people as he can.

I remember once, when I was a child of ten or eleven, sitting and crying in my father's lap, trying to explain how difficult it was for me to make friends. He said *You're just a little shy,*

Jackie. I, too, was shy as a kid. All you need to do is smile and introduce yourself to others. It's easy, he said. *It's easy. You can do it.* But it never seemed that easy.

While driving home, my father says he is proud of me, and that this evening is one of the highlights of his life – escorting his daughter on the homecoming court of the university from which he graduated. He thanks me again for asking him, and then asks if I'd like to go out for a bite to eat. I understand what he is trying to do, his desire to prolong our evening together as long as he can. I tell him I'm not that hungry, but if he is then I'll go with him and we can just sit and talk.

We talk at the restaurant until the last patron leaves and the manager informs us it is time to lock up.

November 5, 1984
Wt: 101 lbs.

My soul weeps bitterly upon hearing the news that my beloved piano teacher has died. My soul weeps but for some inexplicable reason no tears are shed on the exterior.

I feel numb with guilt, and the guilt begins to wash over me for all the things I did not say, for all things I did not do, for having so sorely disappointed him, for never fully recognizing or appreciating the role he played in my life or the fact that he is the one responsible for giving me the keys to my music.

I don't take students that young, he told my mother when I was six. By that time, she had begged him for a year to take me on as his pupil. However, he remained firm in his stance.

Yet despite her unheeded pleas, my mother continued to hound him.

"I have nine students, that's it," he said. "No more. They come to me when they're in their teens and have reached an upper-intermediate level. I prepare them for college and their musical careers beyond."

Having accidentally overheard this declaration, I made the quick assumption that he was just a grouchy old curmudgeon and I therefore wasn't all that keen about becoming his pupil.

My mother remained adamant. *Just listen to her play. Just listen once, and if you say no after that, I won't ask you again.*

So at an age where my feet didn't reach the pedals and my hands only spanned the width of several keys, I played for him. The next week I officially became his youngest student ever.

Miguel taught me what music was truly about. He showed me that music was capable of portraying every human emotion, all the seasons of the earth, all the elements of nature, and any spiritual act or private moment within the mind.

Listen, Jackie, listen to how the waves sound, he would say as he prompted me to close my eyes and assume a posture of silence in order to concentrate on nothing other than what he was about to play.

I would get very still and quiet, and listen to the emptiness of his studio. I could hear the faint whir of the wall-unit air conditioner as it cooled my forehead and maintained the perfect tune of the piano strings. Behind me I overheard the labored breathing of his five Chinese pugs settled together like dominoes while snoring in unison on the loveseat.

Miguel would then assume my place on the bench and bow his head before the keys as if in prayer. He then allowed the silence to enter this space where neither one of us spoke. He said that silence was equally a part of music.

I remained relegated to the side chair, comfortable in the silence, unaware that he had already begun to shadow his large hands across the keyboard. And then he would begin to play.

It started out slowly, a rolling melody improvised from a spirit's spark ignited in that very instant. Beginning in the lower register of the bass keys, his fingers lightly floated up and down, up and down in the same rhythm and scale. While my eyes remained shut, I began to sway with the deep melody and, following suit, my imagination began to kick in.

I was drawn back in time to the brown sands of Galveston beach on a hot Sunday afternoon with my mother and father and brothers and sisters. The sand was hot and wet beneath my feet as we searched for sand dollars and hermit crabs along the water's edge, the furthest point at which the waves swept into the sand dunes before giving up and washing back out again into the gulf.

Miguel continues to repeat the melody, the back and forth rocking motion that sways slower in parts and more rushed in the latter. Lost in my memories, I recall standing on that hot sand as the water rushes across my bare feet and kisses my ankles. Cool, salty sea water that makes its sudden entrance before racing back again to rejoin the sea.

I listen to the same steady motion of Miguel's playing and am reminded of the feeling of the waves that day. *Yes,* I realize, *this is the sound of the waves.*

Then abruptly, he changes the tune. This time it's louder, stronger, filled with strength and fury. My eyes remain closed and I recall the greedy seagulls that soared freely overhead as they flew in irregular patterns, searching for food in the murky waters below or from leftovers strewn across the littered sand. As children we would yell out to them. *"Helloooooo. Can you hear usssssss? Hey stuuuuupid bird!!!"* We would call out to them but the instant the words escaped our lips they were lost among the more overpowering roars of the waves pouring in and out.

Yes, this too is how the waves sound.

To me, the difference in melody represents the waves rolling further out in the ocean. Miguel plays and I hear there are many melodies contained within a single wave. There are numerous melodies and harmonies that all play together to the intricate notes within a thick manuscript, a symphony comprised of tens of thousands of water droplets that splay and thrash and roll and repeat. Miguel played the sounds of the waves and for the duration, a forgotten memory was remembered as I was drawn back in time to that day at the beach.

It was in this same manner that he taught me to play the crackling sounds of fire, the discomfort of heat, the rolls of thunder and the peals of lightning. He showed how to connect to the imagination and a source outside myself to produce the promise of sunlight, the freshness of morning, the purity of joy, and the clarity of water. Through his instruction I discovered that everything and anything could be translated onto the keys of a piano: the melancholy of sadness, exuberance of happiness, timidity of fear, and unabashed bravado.

It was during another lesson when he asked me this question: How do you imagine God feels as he looks over the heavens and the earth he created?

I had no immediate response but eagerly anticipated his interpretation, once again played from his unique vantage point. He was about to deliver his own interpretation through musical delivery, by sounding it out on the Knabe. So once again I moved to the side chair and closed my eyes, waiting in silence. He, in turn, took his place on the bench and began to play a soft, soothing melody in the key of E flat.

With my eyes closed and his music playing in the background my mind began to wander into that outer realm until it met with the image of a kindly white-haired gentleman dressed in a white robe and holding a golden staff. Possessing ageless eyes, he stands barefoot atop a magnificent sapphire orb. Yellow light shrouds his body and a kindly understanding light radiates from his clear blue eyes. There is no mistaking in this imaginary picture that He cares deeply for those under His watch. Sounds create an image, an image that my imagination takes and runs with, pondering all possibilities.

Unlike most instructors of his caliber, Miguel never believed in following a set order of musical progression. He never believed any piece of music was too difficult or too advanced. He recognized that if a student latched onto a piece of music he or she loved, that it would be played with a singular force unique to personal style.

And now he is dead. The opportunity is lost and I cannot thank him for all the things he taught me which were so much more than just music. I cannot tell him that he was more of a grandfather than mere instructor, that he was a godsend who helped stabilize an otherwise shaky earlier existence. I cannot apologize for having disappointed him so deeply by quitting lessons long before I should have. He warned me that my walking away from the lessons would revoke any hopes of a career as a concert pianist. I knew even then the high hopes he had pinned on my future, his prized pupil, but I walked away anyway, realizing, at the age of fourteen, that this was not the career I wanted. I walked out of his studio and out of his life with the cavalier attitude of youth that makes the erroneous assumption that everyone will live forever. I also made the assumption that he knew how great my love for him was.

It is because of this man that I have my music, and now he is dead. And there are no words for the guilt or sorrow I feel. Another whom I have failed. There are the no words to summon the tears that will not shed, tears I must shed, nor are there words to summon the ability to say goodbye. There are so many things I wish I had said, situations I wish I had handled differently to show him I loved him.

He never let me down, but I let him down terribly. I can never forgive myself.

I cannot say goodbye to this man I so loved. I cannot tell him that I will see him again one day in heaven. I refuse to part with that which I now realize was so life-giving during a time when I desperately needed something that filled my soul. Something that offered life so freely without asking for anything in return. I cannot bear to think that he who took me in at so young an age and gave me the keys that opened the door to the magic of music is now gone, never to return. I shake my head, arguing with death, arguing with his fate, berating myself for not telling him I loved him or apologizing for disappointing him. It is too late. I cannot say goodbye to him.

My mother, dressed in black, asks why I am not dressed for the funeral. I tell her I cannot go.

November 10, 1984
Wt: 103 lbs.

I meet Mimi at our favorite restaurant. We are regulars here, warmly greeted upon the arrival of each of our many visits. We are shown to our usual table where our regular waiter says he'll put in an order for margaritas.

After we place our order, my grandmother lights a cigarette. She is unusually quiet this evening, not at all in her usual joking manner. Something weighs on her mind. She takes another sip of her margarita and licks the salt from her lips. The strong tangy aroma of tequila at once fills the surrounding air. She makes no comment when I order a salad void of any meat or cheese. Dressing on the side. She never comments on my eating habits. She never gives me strange looks or glances of disapproval, and because of this she is safe, a safe presence in which my guard can somewhat relax.

"I want to tell you something but I'm not sure how to begin," she says.

I take another sip of my margarita. The tequila is strong. I smile to myself and think about how odd a pair we must seem. Grandmother and granddaughter who meet twice a week at this same restaurant for drinks and dinner, who enjoy each other's company like best friends.

"Shoot," I say. There is no threat in her voice. There never is, and because of this she is safe.

She sighs. "Well, it's like this. Everybody's mad at you. Everybody's mad and they're concerned and they don't know what to do to help you."

"Everybody?" I ask. "Who exactly is *everybody?*"

"Your family," she replies. "Your dad, your mother. Richard, Leslie, Abigail, Daniel. They're all extremely concerned about your not eating. They're worried about how thin you've become. They want you to eat. They want to help you but nobody knows what do do."

Traces of anger begin to set in, anger that they are talking behind my back, no doubt scheming, no doubt invading my privacy even though there is little, if any, privacy within a large family.

"Why would they be angry that I've lost a little weight," I counter.

She does not smile. She is not amused by my attempted joke. "Jackie," she says barely under her breath, "you and I both know this goes way beyond your losing a little bit of weight. You exceeded your original goal, and that was fine. I was proud of you. We all were. I thought that was the beginning for you, the beginning of what you wanted, the start of your new life. I thought you might even get back some of that self esteem you had lost. But now...." Her voice cracks. "It has gone way beyond that. You barely eat enough to stay alive."

I stare at her, taking in her words, feeling the strain in her voice. Then, for the first time I begin to realize the strain that my not eating has taken on her. It has taken a toll and she has not told me. I know that I have caused my parents pain, but because my grandmother has not said anything, it never occurred to me that I have hurt her as well. If I have caused pain to her then surely I have caused pain to others, others whom I have not been aware. She has not wanted to tell me of her worry. I have caused her pain. I see it in her expression and now I hear it in her voice. This is a dam about to burst. She has kept this hidden from me so as not to worry me further. Guilt Guilt Guilt. I have caused her pain. I do not want to cause her pain. I do not want to cause anyone pain. My insides begin to sink with the realization that I am the cause of so much pain.

She continues. "Back in May, when you came home from school....you lost all that weight and you looked great. But here it is November...and you don't eat anything. You run all the time. You eat nothing, and you're skin and bones. Everybody sees it except you. You really don't seem to fathom just how dangerously thin you are."

"Mimi," I press, "I *do* eat. I eat breakfast. I eat lunch. I eat dinner. I just don't want to gain any of the weight back. I like the way I am now."

The instant this last sentence is uttered, I realize how false it is, and how unconvincing I must sound. The truth is that I am never satisfied with my outer appearance. But that is the least of my dissatisfactions. It is the interior that remains the larger problem. How can I ever begin to explain the thoughts that constantly torment my mind on an hourly basis? Thoughts of *You're fat, you're going to gain all the weight back, you're not good enough...* I tell myself I have it all under control. I control my life via my new-found discipline. I am in control. The discarded girl I despise is nowhere to be found. It is *me* who is in control now and I will stop at nothing to prevent that girl of the past from returning. No one will ever place their controls over me again.

"Look," she says, "I'm not here to harp on you. I'm not trying to make you feel guilty about your family. I'm just telling you this because I'm worried for you. And they're all too worried to talk to you about it. They feel that if they try, if they should mention anything at all about it then the problem will only worsen. We all hate sitting by and watching you self-destruct like this."

Now I am indeed curious as to exactly what everyone has been saying behind my back, what they have been plotting. Plotting behind my back. Them against me. Why couldn't they tell me? Why didn't they talk to me face-to-face? I realize that they cannot because of this invisible wall I have constructed, a forbidden zone lined with rows and rows of barbed wire to prevent others from entering. They cannot say anything to my face because I have prevented them from doing so. They implicitly understand that their trespassing onto forbidden soil could cause any hidden land mines to suddenly explode.

I ask my grandmother what they have said. She makes me promise not to repeat what she is about to say. I give her my solemn word.

"Your mom and dad spoke with that psychiatrist again. Apparently, he informed them that if you continue on in the same manner you'll be dead within a year."

We each take a slow sip of our drinks. Any anticipated merriment to be found in our evening together is now long gone. My mortality. It doesn't seem possible that I will die. Other than the mind, my body feels stronger and healthier than ever before. It is my mind that drives me constantly to the edge of insanity, my mind that begs for relief from the pain of so many things I do not understand. I do not attach any credence to the doomed words of the doctor. After all, what does he know? He can calculate on his little statistic chart all he wants. He can meddle into lives of those whom he knows nothing about and come to his scientific conclusions based upon mounds of information and studies. But he knows nothing of me. He cannot understand what is in this mind, this mind that carries the weight of every perceived negative emotion imaginable. And therefore he is unable to attach any remedy, any cure, any knowledge that can clean this filthy heavy slate and turn my life back around.

Mimi continues. "Your family is worried sick, and they feel helpless to do anything because they are quite aware of your refusal to enter a treatment facility. There's more. They feel you've pulled away from the core of the family, that you're off alone in your own world even though you live under the same roof. They say it is as if you are physically present even though you aren't really there."

Like a ghost.

It is true. I have pulled back. Pulled back into a zone of set determination that refuses food and persists in running five miles a day. But, throughout, I never meant to cause them any harm. I would like to think I'm the kind of person who would never want to intentionally create harm to my family or to anyone else. Yes, I have pulled back. But in my large family where much escapes the eyes and ears and much goes un-discussed, where the focus is on the whole rather than the individual, where my parents are just trying to get done what needs to get done, it never dawned on me that all attention would suddenly shift to focus on a single child.

My grandmother continues. "Richard doesn't think you need to go to a treatment facility. He doesn't think that's what you need."

Leave it to Richard who's always possessed a unique mind and viewpoint, who thinks differently from the pack mentality. I wish his mind were more like my own. If I had Richard's mind, I'd never be stuck in this lost land.

"He doesn't think a treatment center would do you any good. Instead, he mentioned another program, one we'd never heard of. Something called Outward Bound

I laugh out loud. Camping. Not my idea of a good time.

I am only vaguely familiar with the outdoorsy, rigorous, fend-for-yourself 30-day program. Other than that, I do not know the specifics. But one thing is for certain, I have never nor will I ever have any desire to camp outdoors.

"Richard thinks you need a program like this to give you some self-confidence. He feels you don't have any sense of what you are able to accomplish, of the strengths comprised within. He says you don't realize about yourself what the rest of us do. He wants to find a program that will re-instill this lack you so desperately need."

It's an interesting thought, one I hadn't before pondered. Strengths within? Capabilities to accomplish anything? Am I guilty of not realizing that I can accomplish something? I don't even know what these strengths are. I'm not even sure of what I want to accomplish.

My grandmother continues. "Richard didn't say it had to specifically be Outward Bound. But that's the general idea. Something that will give you a feeling of accomplishment and self-esteem. That particular program was just the first thing that popped into his mind."

Accomplishment and self-esteem. I find it humorous that he would think that. And yet, on the other hand, I am impressed that he has actually put in the time and consideration with regards to me. Sickly enough, I even feel a little flattered by the unwanted attention.

Something else nags at me, and I say, "I don't understand why they're mad at me."

She replies, "Honey, I don't think they're really mad at you. They're mad at the situation, at themselves for not being able to help you. It's every parents need to help their children, for your siblings to want to help a lost sister. They want to help but are at a loss."

November 13, 1984
Wt: 103 lbs.

Out of nowhere, I suddenly recall two incidences that I had forgotten about. Two faces that had been erased from my memory until one recent evening when I am running. I had forgotten, but now I remember.

The first was a camp counselor named Kendall. After she was introduced to our seventh grade girls' cabin, I stared at her in astonishment as if she were a child much younger than myself. Her legs were matchsticks and her head perched atop a tissue of flesh so thin it seemed it would easily snap off should she lean either too far to the left or the right. She wore oversized blue jean overalls, little girls clothing, and in no way did she resemble a young woman of nineteen. With her slight frame and lack of shape she seemed a fragile child oblivious to the ways of the world.

Whispers among the other counselors convened when Kendall was not around. There was an aura of mystery surrounding this childlike creature that the rest of us campers did not understand and were not privy to. She never ate in the dining hall. She never showed her face at pancake breakfasts. She wore a mask that lacked any expression. No joy formed in her eyes. No smile ever crossed her lips. She wore long pigtail braids, a little girl hairstyle. No matter what the time of day, Kendall remained in self-imposed isolation, and could be seen far-off as she power-walked the dusty trails of the surrounding east Texas hillside. She was present only when it was required. But even when she was present, it was as if she was completely vacant.

One morning, Kendall had suddenly disappeared. When we awoke, her bunk was devoid of sheets and blankets, and her trunk was gone. The camp overseer informed us that her grandfather had suddenly taken ill and that she therefore would not be returning. He then introduced us to our new counselor.

The other forgotten face belongs to the dorm leader. Kelly was her name, and she too possessed a vacuous presence

presence during those brief stints when she did emerge within the ranks of twenty-five frantic females. Like Kendall, she too possessed matchstick legs and arms, and a pre-adolescent figure devoid of any curves. She, too, appeared as a little girl not even old enough to enter high school let alone a senior in college with plans to attend a prestigious law school in the fall.

I do not know why the memories of these girls suddenly re-emerge. I have not thought about them for years. I do not recall much about them other than the fact that I clearly remember thinking how odd they seemed, how different they seemed from girls their own age, and how separated from the pack these childlike creatures were.

November 27, 1984
Wt: 102 lbs.

The world is filled with secrets. Secrets that one will never divulge for fear of tarnishing the exterior image and thus messing up a pretty little world. The world is filled with secrets that hurt, kill, destroy and will only magnify the problem should they be revealed.

The far corners of the world bulge at its seams with secrets that no one wants to discuss, that no one will acknowledge, that no one will share, that no one wants to admit.

The world is filled with secrets that blow the helpless little leaves north and south, east and west until nothing is left of their carcasses except for tattered brown remnants of dried, dead cells. The secrets are tucked away and forgotten during the day. However, at night, when one is not awake to diligently guard them, they become unleashed to torment one's subconscious thoughts and dreams, leaving the one who guards the secrets to toss and turn in bed.

The secrets enter the all-knowing mind of the universe and never leave as long as they are kept safe and hidden. As long as the secrets are kept safe, she knows no safety for it forms the nucleus of her identity. It begins to define her soul, shape her outlook, how she views everything and everyone. The secrets distort all views of things material, physical and emotional, and create a world of unrecognizable static, of incessant buzzing that constantly plays upon the mind of she who guards the secrets.

The world is filled with secrets that kill, destroy, maim, mock and torment she who carries the secret. They serve to limit what the person allows herself to do. She pretends to be who she wants to be. She pretends to be who she's not.

The secrets always lie. The bearer of the secrets learns to lie, to pretend, to make-believe to be something she is not, to pretend that all is well in a world filled with lies. She pretends that all is right in her world when, in reality, the secrets continue to feed and grow on the inside. They grow larger and larger, cancerous tumors that eat away at the truth, turning cells of truth of malignant lies. The secrets need to be excised but removing the malignancy will only destroy she who guards the secrets.

The world is filled with lies. Lies about what is important, lies about what our purpose is on earth, lies about who we are and what we are supposed to be.

The world is filled with secrets that are not always isolated. Two people often share the same secret, each fully aware of the other's charge, but neither is willing to talk about it, reveal its contents or even acknowledge its existence. Neither will admit that the secret is real, that the events surrounding the source of the secret are real and did occur.

The secrets silently destroy the one who carries the secret. Any self-esteem or worth is whittled away as the secret silently crushes any goals and dreams she may have had. It destroys that part of the soul that is real and demands to be acknowledged. It cries out to deaf ears that the secret is real, that it did occur, that it happened to me. It seeks revenge, revenge and justice that she knows will never come to pass. The secrets continue to destroy that part of the soul that lies hidden in grief and does not know how to deal with the growing rage or overcome the sadness.

The world is filled with secrets that prohibit the denial of pain, any hurt, and any consequences of these destructive emotions that need be addressed. In its sinister track, the trail of secrets leaves behind the helpless leaves that sway in all directions within the wind. The leaves sway to the east, then further to the west, then more forcefully to the north, high above the ground where the leaves dangle helplessly while staring at the long fall below and wondering how fast they will come crashing down to the ground, and how much it will hurt.

The secrets of the world kill, maim, destroy and viciously attack those who bear the secrets. The secrets warn her of the dire consequences that are sure to occur should the secrets be exposed. The more secrets there are, the more the secrets taunt, until the person is so twisted and tangled within the web of secrets that she can no longer see out. She can no longer see straight or that which is true. The bearer of the secrets begins to discover that the ability to correctly deliberate between right and wrong is lost among a sordid bed of lies.

The secrets assume the identity of the individual and then, slowly, over time, she begins to think like the secrets want her to think. The person believes that if she tells her secrets then her world will be destroyed, that surely no help will come to avail, that nobody will be interested, that everyone will laugh. The secrets repeat this exercise daily to the individual, a daily prayer with which to follow faithfully and remind her of the dire consequences that will meet her fate should she choose to reveal the contents of this secret.

The cells of the secrets magnify into gigantic, smothering THINGS, burdens that become so insurmountable they can never be revealed. The secrets insist that if they were to be revealed, she will suffer ridicule, mockery, ignorance and even hatred. No one will like her, the secrets say. And in this way, the secrets ensure themselves a guaranteed place of eternal protection within her soul.

November 29, 1984
Wt: 102 lbs.

What would it be like if there were no secrets, if I had been able to tell someone everything that had happened, both the good and the bad? Would anyone have listened? Would anyone have cared? Deep inside, I feel there are many who would have both listened and cared. Was it my fear that prevented me from disclosing the truth?

Yes. Adamantly yes.

Now I fear it is too late. I have spun a web so deep there's no way out. There is no way to expose all the things I carry inside: wanting to be thin, wanting to fit in, wanting to know my purpose in life, wanting to know what career to have, wanting to be liked, wanting to not be afraid of men.

I want to not fear relationships with other women, to not always assume they laugh behind my back. I want to know who I am outside of my family. I want to be able to trust men my age rather than fearing they will inflict physical harm. I want the gray clouds to go away. I don't want to feel nervous about everything, the growing anxiety that brings me closer daily to the brink of insanity. I want to know why I'm not more like my brothers and sisters who are so popular and funny, who seem to everything in the world going for them. I want to live in their world instead of my own.

I think others mistakenly assume these things: that I've got my act together, that I know what I'm doing, that I'm sure of myself, that I know what I want out of life. Their expectations of me are high. They assume that because I am thin, tall, blonde, make good grades, come from a good family, that I have it all together. However the reality caters to none of the above. No one can see the intertwined mess of secrets and fears that are with me always. I am the brown leaf that tosses in the wind, waiting to fall and crash onto the sidewalk below.

How did I wind up like this, with all the world has to offer, from a good family that loves me? How did I wind up making an utter mess of my life?

Isolation is my own choice. But is it really a choice, or rather the invisible secrets that taunt me into keeping to myself, from revealing more than I should, from revealing more than I am capable of? The secrets taunt me, warning that if I were to open up and show all the secrets I've stored inside for so long, that the floodgates will open and the waters will wash me away. Away from my family. Away from my friends. Away from those few precious things I trust and believe in. They will wash me away forever into the sewer where nothing is ever retrieved.

I live in a world of secrets where I pretend to be that which is expected. Perfect. I pretend to be society's ideal image, the object of perfection, because inside I do not know what I want, who I am, or what I am capable of accomplishing. I live in a world of secrets because I do not feel adequate enough to partake with the rest of the world and drink from the same cup of life that they do. I live in a world of secrets because if I were to reveal what is truly inside, no one would believe it.

I live in a world of secrets because of scars that won't heal, and because they have become a part of whom I am and thus determine how I view myself. I live in a world of secrets because it is easier than telling those I love the truth, the truth of what happened to me, for fear they will desert me just like the Mean Girls. I live in a world of secrets because I do not want anyone to see how dirty I am, the shame I carry with me on a daily basis because of a grown man who hurt me when I was a little girl. I live in a world of secrets because inwardly I feel that maybe I deserved to be hurt, that perhaps my predestined fate as a child was to suffer and suffer alone. After all, isn't that what was taught in parochial school – that Jesus delights in our sufferings? Perhaps I deserved to be hurt because I was unworthy and bad and dirty. This was the image projected back at me, and I believed it.

I live in a world of secrets because I do not want to be that bad, dirty, unworthy little girl.

December 5, 1984
Wt: 100 lbs.

I have decided to major in economics. The irony is that it was the one class in high school in which I made a 'D', and even that was a 'take pity on her' last-minute raise from an F. In the innocent years of high school where the prime focus rested upon what to wear to the weekend party, I was unable to fathom the most elementary of basic economic principles.

It is ironic how a different stage of one's life has the ability to see through a veil that was blackened before, bringing topics and issues to light as clearly as if we'd understood them all our life. Suddenly, the field of economics has clicked for me.

Whereas before, I attributed my inability to grasp these concepts taught during high school on the ineptness of the instructor, one with thirty years of experience and who held a Ph.D. Now I realize it was I who was inept for not being able to grasp the full value and meaning of competition in a free society.

"But why do we need competition?" I asked innocently, in the second semester of my senior year. "We're all equal," I rationalized, feeling such pride at my obvious intelligent and enlightened viewpoint that I imagined could be akin to that of a guru on the subject. "Maybe if we could all just help each other out a little more."

The class erupted in laughter, and I too joined in the ebullient mood. It was neither mockery nor chastisement, the laughter of my peers, but rather the ongoing theme of our high school experience, which was to find humor in anything.

Marcia Kominsky, who sat directly at my right, nodded her head in wholehearted agreement. Then others followed her lead, until half the class was nodding in agreement and in direct opposition to what the instructor had attempted so futile to illustrate. The class was in unanimous agreement – competition had no place in our lives. It was an archaic feature of society.

Mrs. Hancock removed her glasses from her nose, placed her manual on the desk and grasped each side of her waist with her free hands. She stared across the room at each one of us, seeing our earnest expressions and audacious presumptions that we knew better than her.

"People," she began, "I can't believe what I am hearing. Don't any of you realize that this country was built and fostered through the spirit of competition? That we enjoy what we have today only because of the spirit of competition? You seem to think that competition is a bad thing. It is, in fact, quite the opposite."

Now here it is three years later and not only has my mindset completely altered from those earlier beliefs, but I grasp now what I could not then. Is this what time does — take you on a winding road through one experience after another until you finally reach a place of understanding where those things previously non-understandable begin to bloom and blossom right under one's nose?

Did I really not view the high school experience as competitive? Perhaps I did although if this was the case, my fiercest rival was probably myself.

December 9, 1984
Wt: 100 lbs.

At school, Andrew takes one look at me and says with concern, "Gray clouds again, Jackie?" It is not a question but rather, a statement.

After he says it, I feel naked, exposed. I go off by myself. I do not want to see anyone. I do not want to talk to anyone. That single question makes me feel more exposed than ever.

But Andrew is gentle soul who always has a kind word for everybody. If he said this, it is only out of concern. Still, the fact remains that he can see the invisible clouds that weigh so heavily in my mind. He can see it. He is the first person to ever say this.

How did these clouds ever attach themselves to me? Why won't they go away? There seems to be no answer, no relief. The only time the clouds do vanish is when I run. I run every day, for weeks without a break. I know that a day without running translates into the clouds worsening. And so I run. An hour a day that provides the only relief from the clouds. It is the only time when I feel free, period.

Every morning when I awake, the clouds are back, dulling my senses, fighting with my insides for their continued reign of domination. The voice inside constantly struggles with the clouds. She silently screams for them to go away, to leave her alone, to show mercy by providing even momentary peace.

I cannot control the clouds. I cannot control when they provide for brief periods of clarity or when they decide to pile up, one atop the other, in a hailstorm. I am tired. I am so tired of struggling with these clouds. I am also tired of worrying about gaining weight. I am so tired of worrying about everything. I do not have the mental strength to continue like this for another year. I am going to collapse. I am going to collapse underneath all this weight.

December 29, 1984
Wt: 99 lbs.

My eating and running habits have affected Leslie. No one else says anything. Leslie doesn't say anything about it either. But I can see her concern. She does not want me out of her sight. She wants to run with me in the evenings. She meets me at the door when I come home from work. Leslie is worried, but she does not say she is worried. For the first time in our lives, we begin to form a friendship as adults, casting aside the pettiness of our youth with funny forgiveness, like the time she used a permanent market to scribble across the forehead of my Madame Alexander doll, and that time when I forced her to kiss Steve Simpson on the lips.

She does not nag me to eat, but she wants to go out, alone, just the two of us, to restaurants where we can sit and chat and drink margaritas. I tell her about Julian, about missing him, about the humiliation. She just sits and listens. I tell her that I never think I will love someone that way again. She listens to everything I say. I tell her about the babysitter. She just listens. She listens in a way that wants to hear more.

I now worry that by confiding my secrets into her trust, that I will somehow transfer the secrets that could potentially harm her as they have harmed me. I do not know whether it is right to tell my secrets, or whether I should continue to keep them contained within.

December 30, 1984
Wt: 99 lbs.

Growing up, our neighborhood was filled with families and children who rode their bicycles barefoot way past dark. Most of the mothers were stay-at-home moms raising anywhere from three to ten kids, most of whom attended the same parochial school. Station wagons were parked in every driveway when not making the endless rounds of errands, carpool, tennis lessons and grocery shopping. Between the sweaty children and their successful parents, there were many savory characters within our neighborhood, and it was a happy place to grow up.

But there was one mother who seemed a bit different from the others. She did not play in tennis matches with the other moms or swim at their country clubs. Sometimes she would visit my mother. I think she liked the company. But they weren't the kind of friends to sit and talk for hours on end. She liked the Steinway in our living room. Her visits usually came while my mother was cooking dinner. It was during these times that she would head for the living room and settle behind the ivory keys. For the next hour or two, she graced our home with the music of the classics, Broadway tunes, songs from the thirties and forties. My mother prepared the meatloaf and tater tots, spurred on by these live concerts.

Then one day she died. It was the first time I had heard of the term suicide.

Immediately following the funeral, Leslie became ill. She stayed home from school for a week with stomach pains, unable to move, not responding to over-the-counter medications. Then she stayed home a second week, and then a third, until my mother took her to yet another specialist who, like the previous M.D.'s, were unable to reach a conclusive diagnosis. At this point, my sister's illness was a mystery to everyone.

Finally, my mother began to put two-and-two together, and one afternoon sat at Leslie's bed side and asked my sister why her stomach hurt so much.

Leslie said that Mrs. Brackenwell had died because she was so sad. And my sister, cognizant that my mother also experienced bouts of sadness, did not want her to succumb to the same fate.

Summoning all forces of subconscious willpower. my sister had glued herself to my mother's side for as long as she could, to keep watch, to guard, to ensure that nothing bad would happen.

Now it is as if I am watching history repeat itself as my sister singularly attempts to revive my will to live.

January 17, 1985
Wt: 99 lbs.

Leslie went back to school and I miss her. It's so lonely here without her.

January 24, 1985
Wt: 100 lbs.

Ten minutes before the Rice library closes for the evening, I stuff my backpack with my notebook and economics book. At the exit door, a student employee wearing glasses and a plaid shirt stops me. I see him several times a week when he checks out my library books. However, this is the first time he has spoken to me.

"Uh, Miss?" he says sheepishly, motioning me aside. He retrieves a folded piece of loose leaf paper from his shirt pocket and hands it to me. "There was a guy in here earlier. He already left, but wanted me to give this to you."

My face flushes as I reach for the note and then hurriedly make my way through the exit, out into the dark, quiet courtyard. When I am safely in my car with the doors locked, I hold the note and, in the darkness, can barely make out the cursive words written in green ink: "For the Girl in Green", a reference to my emerald-colored t-shirt. I carefully open the mystery paper that has been meticulously folded on the diagonal at least five times, probably the handiwork of an engineering major.

The handwriting is concise and elegant with strong, elongated pen strokes. I begin to read.

"For whatever it's worth, I am a new student here, having recently transferred back from Columbia. I have not had time to make new friends yet. I noticed you studying in the corner and wanted to say something to you, to introduce myself, but you appeared involved in your work. I would like to take you to lunch if you have time. Here's my phone number. Jeff."

I re-read the note several times before starting the engine and heading home. I know I should feel flattered. Instead, I feel exposed. I do not know what to do. I do not know how to handle the flattery or the invitation.

January 26, 1985
Wt: 98 lbs.

The note stays in my purse where it is re-read again a dozen more times. I wish I were brave enough to call him. But I have already considered the possible outcomes, all of which are, in my mind, negative. What if he hated me? What if I hated him? What if I got stuck in a restaurant with him and could not escape?

No doubt some form of judgment would occur, and that I cannot control.

I cannot face it. I wish I had some form of control. This is too out of control. I cannot contact him and make any arrangements. I cannot control any of it. This note has thrown me into yet another spiral of feeling out of control. Now because of my ineptitude, surely he will think I didn't like his note, that I didn't appreciate his noticing me. No doubt he'll think the worst, and all because I am unable to control this situation. I cannot go to a restaurant with a stranger, into a restaurant full of food I will not eat, and place myself in the midst of a conversation of which I do not know the outcome.

His note is relegated to my secret box of saved things.

February 5, 1985
Wt: 97 lbs.

I have hurt my family. I have hurt them in ways one cannot see, in ways not physical, in ways invisible to the eye. The hurt I have caused would go undetected by a battery of blood tests or the readings from an MRI. I have not hurt them like a bully picks on the helpless, or a murderer kills. But I have hurt them by my attempts to improve myself. I have hurt them because my attempts to improve myself have destroyed everything.

I have hurt them by not eating and by adhering to the most rigid of diets. Maintaining three-hundred calories and running five to seven miles a day without a break in willpower has hurt them. I have hurt them by maintaining the belief that I am fat as a cow even when they shake their heads in disbelief and argue that it is not true. However, I need only take one look in the mirror to see that it is indeed true.

I have hurt them by cocooning myself within the walls of impenetrable solitude and rejecting all of their offers of help.

In my mind, I rationalize that I am progressing, moving forward, achieving, and attaining the ultimate symbol of perfection. I strive every waking minute to cultivate and hone this symbol. My body and mind are so conditioned to my routine, to the eating habits, to the running, that it is no longer difficult as it was when all of this first began. I no longer feel as hungry as when I first started the diet. The muscles in my calves and thighs no longer ache with the newness of exercise. My mind has taken over all previous habits and now steers on auto-pilot. It regulates when I will eat and when I will stop eating. It reminds me when it is time to run and when all of the daily calories have been exercised away. It tells me when to study and when to sleep and when to go to school and when to go to work. I think I have come far through this discipline, but perhaps the reality is that I have only gone as far as the distance between Dallas and Houston.

I have hurt my family because I do not eat meals with them. I have separated myself from them. I do not laugh much anymore either. There was once a time when laughter reigned. I miss that part, and I know my family misses it too. I do not feel a part of them and they, in turn, realize just how much I have pulled away. I have hurt my parents who bite their tongues and do not say anything and now wear worried frowns and are at a loss for words whenever I am around. I have hurt my sister who seems the most worried of all. I know this is true and yet I cannot tell her that I acknowledge her worry. I cannot reach out to her or open myself up for her to be able to truly reach out to me like she wants to.

I have hurt my family because I have locked myself deep inside the recesses of skin and bones and muscles and ligaments and tendons. I am locked so deep within myself that I have forgotten how to re-emerge into their realm and be a part of the family again. I do not know how to escape from these prison walls I have built. I have hurt my family by creating a situation that has become an ugly reality, one that imprisons and holds me tight within, never allowing for even the tiniest bit of relaxation from its firm grip.

I have hurt them because they do not know what to do, because of this remain terrified. They live in a constant state of bewilderment and helplessness. They blame themselves for whatever they feel they must have done or whatever it is they couldn't control or whatever it was that lured me into this tangled web of all-around deceit. They blame themselves even though they are at a loss as to the exact causes of this web.

I have hurt them because I lie and they know it. I lie that I'm not hungry and I lie that I'm doing fine. I lie that I'm not exhausted and I lie that my life has never been better. I lie that I've never been happier and I lie that I have everything under control. They know I am lying but I would rather lie than admit the truth as to how I really feel.

I have hurt them because they do not know whether I am trying to punish them or whether I am just punishing myself. No one seems to know how the need to control got so out of control, and so they blame themselves. They blame themselves because they do not want to hurt me. They know I am in pain and they do not want to add further to it.

I have hurt them because I have disrupted and scarred the dreams they had for me. All they have worked for, the sacrifices they have made to put all of us through private school. One sunny day they sent their eldest daughter off to college and the next day she returned home and was never the same. She returned home scarred, with a random, unknown, intangible malady that denied any food or nutrition, and introduced an inexplicable blockage on her path of growth that prevented her from maturing into the woman she was meant to be, the woman her parents dreamed she would become.

I have hurt them because at this point in their lives, my parents should be able to see the light at the end of the tunnel, the nearing years when their youngest child finally graduates from college. The focus should be on the nearing destination when all of their children will finally be out of the nest, out on their own, building lives and careers and homes, finding mates and securing the rights for future grandchildren. Even with the financial burden of college, this should be some of their best years, the final years of enjoying their children at home, enjoying the fulfillment of watching them mature and grow into young men and women. They should be enjoying the pride of their accomplishments in child-rearing, all they accomplished together in raising five children. I have hurt them because I have robbed them of this, have taken away their joy and excitement, have decimated the dreams they had for me.

I have hurt them because I have replaced this home with worries that did not before exist, with problems for which there seems to be no explanation, with problems that they know and believe could realistically lead to the death of their child. I have hurt them because the psychiatrist told them that should my dietary habits and mental attitude not improve soon, I will be dead within the year.

I have hurt them because I have cut short the dreams they had for me, dreams of watching their eldest daughter receive her college diploma, then venture out into the workforce and eventually marry and have children. I have hurt them because now they see none of this happening for me. Now when they look at me, they see a future that includes a wooden coffin and a tombstone. They see a future that involves making funeral arrangements followed by the endless grief of losing a child so unexpectedly and needlessly.

I have hurt them and they did not deserve any of this. This is my entire fault, of my own doing, of my own hurt and pain. This is the result of my striving for perfection in the world in which I live where nothing is perfect.

I have hurt them by introducing this burden they do not understand and have no control over. They try to fathom exactly what could have occurred to cause such a downfall. I have hurt them because no matter what I do to try to make it up to them or show them that I love them, I cannot find the words or the voice. That voice, silenced so long ago, no longer exists.

I have hurt them because before there were seven of us. Now there are six plus one-on-the-side, the family member who suddenly and inexplicably extricated herself from the central unit and went off into a world of her own. Lost within her thoughts and beliefs and sadness and fears and self-doubts and starvation and endless running. There is no union between one side and the other no matter how hard each side tries or how firmly each wills it to happen. The two sides are now separated by the gate of food control.

They will do anything, anything at all to be able to understand what went so horribly wrong whereby the one-on-the-side now starves herself with one foot in the grave.

I have hurt them through my inability to control the situation. I realize that they are the last remaining people I can count on, those who love me no matter what, no matter how much I have hurt them. I do not know how to deal with the guilt I feel. They do not think I care or that I am aware of the pain I have caused, but nothing could be further from the truth. I care so much and am so aware of all the pain I've caused. I wish I could just crawl into a hole somewhere in the middle of an unnamed, unmarked desert and die, where I could be forgotten, as if I'd never existed. And in my place I would appoint the perfect girl, the perfect beautiful smart intelligent female who is capable of anything. Someone who would be the perfect big sister, the perfect daughter.

I have brought into our home an invisible demon that no one can see, hear, smell, taste or feel. A demon that no one can determine from where it came or why it appeared. Or why it won't leave. A demon that waits silently, menacing, adding burden upon burden to my unsuspecting and unequipped parents and siblings. The demon is there in the morning, there at night. It is there during the quiet hours of slumber. It remains within the house all the time. It never goes away.

I have hurt them because I have introduced this demon into our home and watched helplessly as it destroys them while at the same time it destroys me.

I have hurt them because I do not know how to solve this problem.

February 10, 1985
Wt: 99 lbs.

It seems there is only one who is not angry with me: God.

This creator, the one I have known since I was a little girl, is far different from the one taught in grade school. He is different from the terror preached in Sunday sermons. He is not at all the stern judge waiting to impart tough sentences, nor is he the Creator as taught in my college courses who adheres to the rigidness of man-made rules for a purpose never of his essence.

Our relationship has never included any of these things.

I talk to him as my friend, my mentor, one who never judges me. He is safe. He is safe to talk to because despite all that I have been taught, the terror of his eternal reign, this is not the friend who has revealed himself to me. Throughout our discourses, there are no drawn battle swords, no threats of terror or damning judgment, no discussions of guilt or blame. The God I talk to is not that who I was taught about in school. It is the God I know in my heart.

Every night when my head falls against the downy softness of my pillowcase, I talk to him. I tell him about my struggles, about the running, about the dieting, about the gray clouds and the worries and the fears. I tell him everything I've ever been through. I tell him everything, and in return He says he already knows. He comforts me with the implicit awareness that he already understands.

I talk and He listens, and sometimes He talks and I listen. I ask Him if it is true that Jesus delights in our suffering. I am afraid to listen to His answer for fear that it will be true, and that this would then mean a God that I did not know at all. If Jesus did delight in our suffering, then would he have delighted over how an evil man caused such suffering in my life? Would he also delight over the role the Mean Girls played?

Lately I have been falling asleep during the middle of my meditations. When I awaken, I apologize for being so rude. It seems as egregious an offense as taking a snooze during a board meeting with the Chief Executive Officer. However, immediately upon apologizing, I am filled with an otherworldly feeling, a message delivered more as a gut feeling, that assures me I have nothing to fear as far as He is concerned. He tells me that it was He who delivered me into the much needed slumber, that He willed me to sleep because He knew that what I needed most at that time was rest.

I tell Him how sorry I am for hurting my mother and father, for worrying my brothers and sisters. I apologize for making such a mess of my life. I apologize for everything. I ask him if he can make the gray clouds go away, if he can free me of the anxiety. With my eyes closed in the communion of silence, the same mind image always appears. I am kneeling on a white marble floor next to the gold throne in which He sits. But He never allows me to remain on the floor for long. He knows the floor is too cold. He gently reaches for my arms and draws me onto his lap where I will be more comfortable, where He can hear more clearly what I have to say, where He can love me closer. I am enveloped within His flowing white robes and His soft voice. I am enveloped within a love like I have never felt on earth. It is a love of pure acceptance and acknowledgment for all that I am. I remain seated on his lap while he rubs my back and helps to calm me. Even with the many pressing concerns of the world, He has plenty of time for me, all the time I need. He assures me that everything will be all right. He asks me to return to Him again and again.

February 28, 1985
Wt: 100 lbs.

I do not like to eat in the school cafeteria where my salad outfitted with a single tomato slice and exempt of anything else including dressing seems to be the object of much curiosity. *No wonder you're so thin,* others say to me as they first surmise the scant plate on my tray then quickly assess me from head to toe.

I only eat there when I'm famished or when the isolation of going home alone is so great it is worth the humiliation of exposure.

March 3, 1985
Wt: 96 lbs.

Bone tired. I have never felt so worn-out. Yet despite the chronic fatigue, not a single day is allowed to pass without running at least four miles.

The route never wavers as its distance has been calculated as meticulously as that of the daily caloric intake. The familiar path starts at my driveway, proceeds down the block and then through the neighborhood. Every inch of pavement along the way is an assuring familiarity, as are the paint colors of each home I pass and the family canines that graze their beds of St. Augustine. Even the pink and white azaleas whose mouthy blossoms defy the reproach of the late winter months add an additional twinge of certitude that completes the course of this daily footage. I am familiar with every car parked in each driveway, which curbs retain the most water following a heavy downpour, and every street sign and mailbox along the way. These are the things that do not change.

The longest part of the stretch begins as I exit the neighborhood onto Westheimer Road, the major thoroughfare that connects the city's east side to the west. I travel the sidewalk heading east, going with the flow of traffic. It is a narrow pathway shielded beneath the grace of sweetened magnolias and faithful oaks. Cracked and uneven, the sidewalk demands my full attention to prevent any stumble or fall.

During rush hour, this path is overcome with the smell of oil and gasoline from the bustling Ford dealership across the street. Exhaust from the heavy traffic combines with stifling humidity to create conditions non-conducive for outdoor exercise. Congestion begins to pile heavily, leaving those of homeward destinations with little choice other than to accept that which time and patience allows. The car salesmen wave at me as I pass. I am a daily fixture with which they can set their clocks to. I wave back and then turn up the volume of my Walkman. The loud bass and drums of Earth, Wind & Fire blast through the speakers, and my steps fall in sync to the rhythm of the fast-paced beat.

To the right of the dealership sets the Jack In The Box where the thick smell of greasy burgers and fries combined with that of fried clams and spicy wings from the KFC next door conjure a curious whiff attributed to that unique formulaic blend found in urban vials. Within inches of each other's bumpers, exports and imports press onwards at a slow steady climb. The sun dwindles low within its smoky canvas just before making its evening descent, and a wave of tangerine ribbons cascades into the looming gray horizon. It is that transitional point of each day that can neither be defined as precisely day nor night. One by one, a brigade of headlights begin to flicker on, sending streams of ivory shadows to illuminate that which is yet barely perceptible.

Suddenly an earsplitting blare of a locomotive bellows belligerently in the distance. The reverberating blast thunders again even louder a second time as the machine rolls forwards towards Westheimer in steadfast fury. Its force is undeniable as its deep vibrations extend to the very core of the sidewalk's foundations, and energizes the air with radiating atoms that build an invisible chaos. The power of the train's sudden intrusion claims its rightful force over man, creatures and even traffic.

I am a half-mile away from where the tracks cross, too far away to beat the train. I slow my pace.

Seemingly from out of nowhere, the normally dormant crossing lights suddenly come alive as their ruby eyes begin to blink boldly. On and off they signal – red, stop, red, stop – in the ensuing darkness to caution incomers. Then an ornery buzzing noise erupts, this time from the crossing gates as its zebra-like painted posts slowly begin to lower their weight to block the oncoming traffic. Disregarding these early warnings, several impatient drivers slyly maneuver around the impassible trenches to the east side of the road.

Having rounded the bend, the train comes within full view, a darkened tunnel that glides surreptitiously into the eclipse of the surrounding shadows. As it nears, its deep bullhorn once again bellows, and the loudness causes me to stiffen and cringe.

The train begins to pass before me, pulling an endless congregation of steel compartments. A thick coat of rust colors the exterior of each, leaving the discarded remains of an incomprehensible hodgepodge of numbers and letters. I stand on tiptoe in attempt to determine how far off lies the caboose, but there is no end in sight. Years of experience living near these tracks instinctively tells me this is going to be one very long train. The wait will be even longer.

I glance at my Swatch and consider re-tracing my steps back home. That would at least allow for the extra miles needed without getting too far behind in time. Tonight, there is much reading to accomplish and several lengthy assignments to write. There is no time to waste, and therefore I cannot wait needlessly at these railroad tracks. But it is imperative that I run, to maintain the daily distance that keeps this weight at bay. The only means by which to ration time is to re-trace my path. As of now, going forward is impossible. The only feasible path points backward.

As I consider this sole option, I begin to realize that by doing so, I would be running back against the traffic, against all those people sitting in their parked cars, with nothing to look at and nothing to do other than to stare at a runner.

When I gaze back as far as I can see into the dimmed view, there spans long rows of shadowed cars whose blinding headlights radiate in my direction. My mind persists with tortuous thoughts as I begin to envision what these drivers might be thinking, what their perceptions might be of the jogger in the dark. I know it is crazy to think these thoughts that pit one against the other, but these are the thoughts that continually plague my mind. Why would anyone even waste a thought on such a temporary reversion? I cannot help thinking these thoughts. Their gymnastics somersault and tumble constantly in the playground of my mind. I feel judged by others at all times, even by these throngs of anonymities who sit waiting in the obscured shadows. The judgments never end. I will never be good enough. I will never meet anyone's expectations. I don't even meet my own expectations.

With regards to the collective judgments of the murky masses, I quickly arrive at a conclusion. Without a doubt, all is negative. They will form their negative judgments against one they don't even know merely by what they may so briefly see darting alone in the darkness. A mass of anonymities who simultaneously cast their mental votes in the unattainable ballot box. All who will evaluate that which they do not even know, thereby reaching the unanimous conclusion: negative bad, unworthy. The list of negatives continues indefinitely. Despite the chill in the air, beads of perspiration begin to soak my forehead.

I want to run back home, but I cannot. I cannot further the humiliation of running against the many faces who pass judgment. There are too many of them. Too many drivers and too many minds and too many judgments. All those people staring and forming their negative opinions. I cannot run back. I cannot place myself in a position where I am the object of others' stern judgments. I am trapped.

I tug the baseball cap down to further shield my face. I do not want them to see me. I do not want them to see the panic in my eyes. No one shouts anything, no one says anything but despite this, I feel the power of their stares. I feel the intensity of their stares as they sit idly behind their steering wheels waiting for the train to pass. I wish there was another exit route, an escape from the stares and the judgments.

All of a sudden, like a pre-emptive message from the United Broadcast System, I have reverted back in time and now stand at the front of the classroom facing the Mean Girls. They point and jeer and throw scissors at my face. They are all laughing at me and their laughter sizzles the shallow layers of epidermis and fries the cells of my brain that only wants one thing: to get out. 'Look at her clothes,' they laugh even harder. 'Look at her hair. Look at her skin. Worthless. Unusable. Ridiculous.'

There is nowhere to turn. Nowhere to go. I must stand here at the stake to be burned further by their hateful rejection.

I want to hide but there is no hole in which to crawl. There is no moth-eaten gray coat in which to wrap myself. There is no welcoming symphony of dead musicians this far away from the comfort of my piano bench. The fortress doors are locked for the evening. There is nowhere to hide. No escape route lies anywhere to be found.

There is nothing in this nothingness, and I am stuck here in front of this unending train with nowhere to turn. There is no alternative other than to wait along with everybody else and be the suspicious target of their peering eyes.

My heart races as fast as that of the train that continues to power mightily before me. There is no way out. Will there ever be a way out? Or will I continue to run each time the mouth of the past outstretches its hungry jowls to remind me of what once was?

I try to steady my nerves upon the realization that the only alternative is to wait. Wait and pretend that I'm not here. Pretend that I am not standing in front of the Mean Girls in cringed expectation of the next onslaught. I must try to breathe slowly and will my mind to wander elsewhere. I turn up the volume of my Walkman to drown out the surrounding exterior and alleviate the chaotic combustion that has gathered in my head. I walk to the bridge that borders the base of the tracks.

Suddenly, even the reeling overture of Gloria Gaynor is drowned out by the intrusive screeching of the train's steel brakes. Metal grinds against metal as the wheels screech and strain against the steel bands of the tracks in attempt to bring the moving force to an abrupt halt. For no apparent reason, the train is grinding to a sure stop. I feel my tension growing, my anxiety loosening on a rampant tear. *No, no, no, please don't stop the train*, is my only thought, my fervent prayer as I silently beg for it to resume its course.

Again I consider re-tracing my steps. This can't be happening. I cannot be trapped here like a deer waiting to be shot and gutted. I turn every which way there is to turn in search of an outlet but my insides sink further to know there is no available course. There is no telling how long the train will be stalled. It could be three minutes. It could be an hour or more. No one knows and my heightened anxiety has now refused to surrender to further negotiation. I must run. If I do not run, I may gain an overnight pound. But I cannot re-trace my steps. I cannot face all those people. I need a way out. I need a way out. There must be a way out.

With my heart pounding and my mind battling the army of mercenary messages, I stand at the bridge, feeling more than overwhelmed. The heat of metal baked in a full day's sun beats against my brow. Glancing into the ditch below, I pretend to be absorbed in something of interest, anything to take my mind off what is now becoming a full-blown panic attack forming within my chest. A vise tightens around my stomach, squeezing it like juice from a Valencia. It has started. The panic attack has started. Everything begins to feel tight. Perhaps if I don't stare at the judgment of the cars, they will return the favor by their not bothering to look at me either. But there is nothing interesting to see in the scattered mess of paper cups, plastic cutlery and cigarette butts that float in the shallow grassy marsh below.

I step back and search for another object on which to focus my attention, anything in which to preserve my near-collapsed nerves. But there is nothing other than the stopped train before me. I am utterly panic-stricken, and my heart is beating so fast it seems it will leap straight out of the bars of my ribcage. Surely this is what it feels to be dying of a heart attack. I clutch my chest and gasp for air. This cannot be happening. I must get out of here. Somehow I must find a way to extricate myself from this situation before I collapse.

It wouldn't be so bad were I not the sole individual standing here, alone and within view of everyone. Alone and exposed. Exposed for everyone to see and for everyone to judge. Exposed out of my control. This situation is out of my control and it feels ugly and dark and gross and stifling and death-like. As was always the case, no control equals pain. I want this to end. I always wanted it to end. But it never ended. I want this to end now.

My chest begins to further tighten and it becomes more difficult to breathe. I cannot get enough air into my lungs. Hyperventilation sets in as I unwittingly begin to take rapid shallow breaths. White spots begin to sprinkle into my vision, further eclipsing an already darkened view. I need water. I need air. I need to get out. I must find a way out.

My skin is sweaty and flushed, and I feel more like an open target than I've ever felt before. An open target awaiting assassination by a splay of bullets and arrows. A target at which others look, stare, smirk, ridicule, mock, torment, and judge. A target condemned for nothing befitting one who so obviously deserves nothing. I do not want anyone to look at me. No eyes are invited to stare. Unwanted glances are unwelcome. I cannot believe I stand once again in an openly-exposed situation that breaches the text of my control.

But there is no pretending. The fear is now heightened to the point where it will not allow for any hidden retreat into the mind. The fear that is so consuming that even the doors of the steel fortress are now beyond my reach. There is nowhere to go, nowhere to hide.

Silent urges cry out from the very core of my being, urges that demand an immediate withdrawal from the horror of this distress, to remove myself from this situation, to remove myself from this agony, this place that causes so much anxiety. Crying out to be released from this shoddy spotlight, my soul screams louder than it has ever screamed before. It screams to be acknowledged. It demands that for once I acknowledge its voice. This time I desperately want to grant it its wish. And yet there is no escape. I cannot quench the cries for I see no means of escape. Despite the cool climate, my insides burn with rage and fire and hell and fury at the unwanted encore of all these fears I have tried to hide and control.

The head of the train has stopped more than a half mile to my left. To my right, there is no sight of the caboose. I am stuck.

I stare at the wheels of the train. Massive silver orbs thick as tree trunks with a singular strength that could effortlessly squash me into a dripping memory of mashed peas. I count them – one, two, three, four, five, six, seven, eight – eight wheels supporting the tonnage of a single cab. The disks do not bear the brutal rust as the rest of the train. Their silvery finish casts an eerie glimmer against the dim surroundings.

As I stare into the wheels, my mind continues to race. There must be a way out. If I do not find a way out, I will certainly die standing here. I examine the compartment helm towering over me. It is too high to scale. I search to the left and then to the right. There is no way out. My mind continues to race. There must be a way out.

Then suddenly, the beginnings of an idea form, a preposterous idea that seems so outrageous I feel it just might work.

Could it work? Is this my way out? Eyeing the cab top to bottom, I wonder if this is indeed the way out. Is this my escape route? I ponder the merits of this hasty plan. Can it work? It has to work. It must work. It is the only feasible alternative.

Crouching low against the pavement, I check the view underneath the cab set directly in front of me. This perch presents a clear view of the east side of the road where even longer rows of those stalled sit in idle waiting. Even through the faint filters of smoke, I see the next traffic light a half mile ahead. The light changes from green to yellow to red, before recycling back to green. All outside commotion seems to suddenly cease and the only sound I hear is the pounding within my chest. On the free side lies trendy Highland Village shopping center with parking lots lined with Mercedes and Jaguars. Window displays flaunt the latest spring attire outfitted upon rubber band-thin fiberglass models.

There is where I long to be, on the other side, the half from this bisected whole that represents the freedom unavailable here. It is the freedom that would melt this addled anxiety and stricken panic, melting solid into liquid that can then evaporate into thin air. It is the side that is my escape, the escape to freedom, the place where no one can judge me and where my own self judgment will abate. It is the side where nobody can hurt me anymore, and where I no longer hurt myself. The other side is where I must be, not trapped here behind this unmovable beast that is the source of so much pain.

Remaining in a crouched position, I estimate the width of the underbelly. It is perhaps ten feet across, maybe more. I would have no trouble fitting underneath its carriage. The trick therefore lies in the ability to crawl fast enough. Can I do it? Can I do it? If I crawl as fast as my knees will carry me, I can crawl straight under, clear to the other side.

I know it will work, just as long as the train does not re-boot the instant I begin to make my move. If it remains in its current passive state, I will be safe, and therefore free. I wonder if it is possible. I wonder if I have the nerve. One fractional move of these mighty wheels will squash me just like those undeserved peas.

I mentally calculate the time it will take. Six, perhaps seven seconds to crawl on my hands and knees across the wooden tracks. As long as everything goes smoothly and I don't get stuck on a nail or have my shoelaces caught in a split piece of wood or my shirt accidentally hinged to the cab's lower belly, then I will be just fine. It's worth a try. It's worth anything to remove myself from this exposure. It's worth the risk to cross over to the side of freedom that awaits just several feet away. I'm sure I can do it. Somehow I will make this work. I must make this work. I have no other choice than to make this work. I can be fast. I can crawl faster than I have ever crawled before. It is worth the risk to be out of the glare of these unforgiving spotlights, away from the fears, away from the fears, away from the fears. I can do this. Just as long as my timing is perfect and the crawl is made within seconds and the train remains idle.

I can do it. I must do it. If I do not, I will die here.

I inch closer to the train, breathing in the fumes of the sifted coal contents contained within. I can smell the animal's metal, the machinery grind of the brakes that ground this creature to a screeching halt. Vapors of metal circulate onto my skin, permeating my pores. The metallic stench pervades the follicles of my hair and turns my taste buds into a palate of bitter aluminum. I need to be out of here. I must get to the other side. I want it so much that I will take this risk. I can do this.

Again I inch forwards, even closer this time, now within inches of the stationary wheels whose shining mirrors reflect my precarious image back at me. They are much wider than I originally anticipated, and appear even more merciless this close up. Do I dare make this crawl? Do I have the guts? Is it worth taking this chance to alleviate this all-consuming anxiety, these fears?

Yes, adamantly yes.

Mentally, I chastise myself for not having already gone ahead and forged the miniscule distance. By now I could have cleared the east side and been on my way, running the needed miles, running away the black bleakness that never leaves my head, running away all the anxiety that riddles my entire body. I inch even closer, within four inches of the wheel. Now I will make my move. Now. I will not think about it any longer. Now. *Please,* I think to myself, *please train don't move.* Now. Go. I silently plead to no one there to listen, *please let me get to the other side.* Now.

Crouching on all fours, I begin to crawl forwards. I lower my head to avoid any clearance. I cannot allow my hair to get caught. The heat grows even more intense the closer I get, but each forward inch of progress equates to that of a mile separated from the past. Gravel pebbles engrave nicks and scrapes on my kneecaps. My hands grasp at sifted rubble. I can do this. I can crawl straight under this train. My shoulder accidentally brushes against a searing hot wheel, and for an instant my grip is lost. I feel a sharp scratch and look down at one knee that is now bleeding. My hands are covered in a blackened film.

"Young lady?" an older man's voice calls out in the darkness. There is no doubt this stranger I do not see is trying to summon my attention. Tepid alarm rings within his voice. Concern. Disbelief. I pretend not to hear him as I tuck my head further and begin to crawl forward.

Just then, the grating sounds of metal once again jar from the forefront, breaking off the lapse of suspended silence. Metal grates upon metal as the brakes jerk on and off to unleash their temporary pause on the tracks. The train makes a jerking motion and then stops just as abruptly. The engine starts up. Fear balls in my stomach as I stumble backwards, feeling several loose strands of hair catch and break against an overhead pole. I land on my backside. The red warning lights begin to flash on and off again as the train prepares to resume its ride. In the distance arises the faint sounding of its horn as its wheels slowly begin to roll forward. The sun has long disappeared and the silver sways of the wheels begin to roll again in unison as it continues its winding path.

April 16, 1985
Wt: 97 lbs.

I have nightmares about the train and the fact that I nearly crawled under it. I awaken in a cold sweat with the realization that I was within inches of ending my life. I know it was a stupid thing to do. In hindsight I realize this. But at the time there seemed to be no other choice. No other choice other than to put myself in a situation where I could have been killed. My mind has submerged to the point where I believe this is my only choice. How could this have happened? How did I seem to wake up one day to find that I had sunk so low, that my mindset had veered so far off the right path? I know it didn't happen overnight. I know this is the result of years of ignoring the problems, years of pretending that the problems didn't matter because I didn't matter.

This did not happen overnight, but what cannot be denied now is the mindset which now shapes my thoughts and forms my daily patterns. It is not the mindset that I thought would have appeared once I lost all the weight. It is not the mindset that nurtures promise but rather, one that instills fear. Nonetheless, it is the result. It is the result of too many years of towing in treacherous waters, ignoring all the warning signs that demanded attention and help.

And now my mindset has reached the point where the pain of anxiety and panic is so overwhelming that I will risk my own life in order to be free from its clutching talons that pierce the core of my soul.

I risked my life in order to escape the fears. I risked my life for the chance to be free of all of this. I risked my life because the pain is so great. The pain is greater than anything else, even the value I place on my own life.

I do not want to die.

I do not want to die but I do not want to live like this any longer. How do I begin to live? How do I begin to truly live?

Can life be lived without all this fear?

May 20, 1985
Wt: 99 lbs.

My junior year is finally over. Only one year left until I graduate, and I still haven't the foggiest clue of what to do with my life. I am scared. I want to stay within the safe confines of school until I know what to do. How do I begin to devise a plan for my life? How can I take control of those things that control me?

If I have been able to control food for this length of time, surely it would seem there are other things within my control.

August 6, 1985
Wt: 101 lbs.

Margaret has rented a 1930's bungalow next door to campus. She asks me to be her roommate. I am so excited. She says the house has a piano, and that she envisions us sitting around it and singing late into the evenings. I am so excited. This could be a new beginning.

She shows me the interior. It is fully furnished with antique pieces of the Victorian era. There is a den, dining room, kitchen, two bedrooms upstairs with a screened-in porch attached to one. The front porch is covered and has a wooden swing. But the best feature of all is the baby grand Yamaha set catty-corner in the living room. It is in perfect tune. Margaret relays how she came across such a find: by playing Irving Berlin for the owner who immediately congratulated her as the new tenant even though there were dozens of others interested in the house. Neither one of us can believe our luck.

I cannot believe this will be my next home. I love it. The owner, knowing we are students, extends a most reasonable rent. We will absolutely love living here. Playing grown-ups in a grown-up house filled with furniture.

We begin making plans for move-in day. My mother says she can't recall the last time she saw me this excited. She is happy for me.

Margaret is fun. She always makes me laugh. We share the same love for music. There is always much to talk about when we are together. I cannot wait to move into the house. Yet, I feel somewhat hesitant, a little nervous about the prospect. I am nervous that somehow I'll wreck this friendship the same way I've done in the past by my eating and running addictions. I don't want this to happen. I don't want any of that to stifle and choke this friendship.

On the other hand, I know that she is aware of my problem. However, she never says anything about it. She doesn't inquire, she doesn't judge me. It is as if she accepts that part of me but at the same time brings out the other facets – the laughter, the humor, the music kinship – that have long been in hiding. There are some people who bring out the hidden parts we don't realize exist.

I cross my fingers and pray that everything will work out because this is one friendship I do not want to lose. For once, I begin to look forward. I can envision myself living here, all the fun we will have. I can envision all the laughter that will take place here, the secrets we will share, the parties we will throw. There is a lot in store here. That I can see.

September 9, 1985
Wt: 102 lbs.

Richard has transferred to school here. For whatever reasons, he has decided to try giving a smaller university a shot. As I expected, he immediately fit in and has made more friends in the first few weeks than I did over the entire past year. How I wish I had one tenth of his charisma that instantly draws others to his side. I am glad he is here even though now I am known as 'Richard's sister'. He makes friends easily, and they are the kind of people I like too – funny, smart, and down-to-earth. I wish I had met all of them last year when I felt so lonely, but I did not because of my shyness, my self-imposed isolation, my addictions that keep my self-contained exile. With him here, it is as if he has opened a door for me, the door to more friendships.

September 18, 1985
Wt: 103 lbs.

My girl friends and I spend the evening drinking frozen margaritas. We lament the fact that Christmas is right around the corner and our bank accounts border upon negative balances. We ponder ways to earn extra money.

As the pitcher slowly drains into our icy glasses, an idea begins to form, tiny seeds that begin to foster a crazy idea. Helene suggests, "Why not form a singing group?"

We ponder the thought just long enough for it to sink in, and then slowly, smiles begin to form all around the table. Wide smiles and bright eyes because we know this is one business that is tailor-made for us. Enthusiasm is rampant as all the pieces quickly emerge, and we begin to piece together the beginnings of our new venture. Yes, why not combine our singing backgrounds and musical skills to form a quartet for the upcoming holiday season. There isn't another group like it in the city. We'll make a fortune.

Immediately, assignments are divvied out. I am in charge of buying all repertoires, Christmas music set to four-part harmony. Helene will organize the marketing and public relations side. Margaret will compile a list of those to whom we will send our announcement, and she also will handle the booking and business end. I will sing alto and play the piano, Helene will sing soprano, and Margaret the second-soprano. We realize the need for a fourth girl to complete the quartet. Helene says she knows the perfect person.

With so much to do within such a short timeframe, we agree to meet again next week to begin rehearsals.

"But wait," Margaret says, "we need a name for the group. What shall we call ourselves?"

With the aid of a second frosty pitcher, dozens of potential names are tossed about for consideration: The Quarter Notes, Christmas Muses, Holiday Greetings. All are stale, not at all what we are searching for. We are about to give it up for the evening and resume this discussion at next week's rehearsal when suddenly Margaret suggests, "What about The Four Calling Birds?

The margarita glasses unite in a toast at the center of the table. Our singing group is born.

September 28, 1985
Wt: 103 lbs.

The running is now up to five miles a day. I jog the mile over to Rice University, run the three miles surrounding the campus, and then head back home. I run more but am eating even less. It doesn't make sense even though I am happy living in the bungalow, thrilled with my new roommate, and am about to embark on this new business venture. I am moving forward but with regards to the food, it feels I am regressing.

My friend, Curtis, who also has never commented on my private habits, has apparently noticed a further decrease in my weight. Because his father is a surgeon, Curtis possesses more than the standard student knowledge regarding health and wellness. He asks me if I eat protein. I tell him no. He says it is important to eat chicken, beans, eggs. My body needs it, he says, and due to the running, I should also consume carbohydrates.

Is he crazy? I think to myself. Those foods contain way too many calories, and are therefore off limits to me.

I do not want him to be mad at me. I do not want my strange habits to estrange my relationship with Curtis because he was my first friend at this school. I talk to him every day. He knows something is wrong, off. He knows it but he doesn't say it. He has never said anything about it. He does not talk behind my back, and I know this because he does not talk behind others' backs. He is safe, and has been from the start. But what good is it to attach oneself only for safety reasons?

There are many things I feel he would say if I allowed it, if I had ever given any indication or green light that this was an approachable topic for me. But it has not been, nor will it ever be. For now, I must satisfy within the safety of those who will just allow me to be.

I know that he knows he has taken a big risk by mentioning these food issues that I should be aware of. I listen, but it is in one ear and out the other. I will not eat anything just because it is supposed to be good for me. Doesn't he see that I am unable to do this? Can't he realize that even the smallest course of what he mentions will unravel everything?

October 6, 1985
Wt: 102 lbs.

We meet four times a week at the bungalow where we rehearse for several hours. The progress is slow as each member learns her separate lines for more than fifty Christmas songs. None of us had an inkling of the magnitude of this undertaking, in particular the time required to combine the harmonies. However, it does not seem like work. There is no tedium. My favorite is the Nun's Chorus from The Sound of Music.

Already we have a dozen bookings, gigs that begin the weekend following Thanksgiving. We can already hear the cash register ringing with the impending proceeds. I plan to buy great gifts for my father and mother and each of my siblings. This will be a good Christmas for my family. This is fun.

October 10, 1985
Wt: 102 lbs.

While reading the business section of the paper, I happen across an advertisement for the City Marathon to be held in

January. Twenty-six miles. I wonder if I could run that far. I wonder if I can run a marathon. I've never run twenty-six miles before. Not even half that distance.

Could I be a marathon runner? Although it seems a far-fetched notion, there is something so unattainable in its elusiveness that makes me want it that much more. I know I could run part of it. But the whole? That's the question. It's as if this is a feat unattainable to the average, like Einstein discovering The Theory of Relativity. Yet thousands participate in the race. If thousands can do it, then surely I, too, might stand a chance given the proper training.

I want to set this goal and see if I could achieve it. If I can, perhaps there will be other goals I can also set and reach.

October 13, 1985
Wt: 101 lbs.

I head for the bookstore in search of a marathon training manual. The sales clerk looks at me funny, as if I don't fit the image or appearance of a long-distance runner. I am dying to know exactly what she is thinking. No doubt she is judging me. She easily locates the book I need.

The training schedules show months of training needed to prepare. As I peruse the pages, I realize that if I were truly serious about running twenty-six miles then preparations should have started months ago. Set intervals of running patterns are suggested, alternating in the earlier months between five and eight miles, and working up to the latter months, just before the race, where longer practice runs include eighteen and twenty-one mile stints. I do not have enough time in my day to pencil in an extra two hours to run. Not between school and studying and violin lessons and music rehearsals.

In addition to the running schedule, there is an entire chapter devoted to diet, a high carbohydrate system designed to fuel the body for long distance. I gaze through the daily menus, shaking my head in disgust as I read the contents for a heavy breakfast, lunch and dinner, including lots of high protein and carbohydrate snacks in between. Already I consume less than a tenth of what is suggested as a proper marathon diet. There is no way in hell I will enforce such a diet. No way. A big bowl of granola cereal with two bananas and a yogurt for breakfast? And that's just for starters. No way.

Still, I wonder if it is possible for me to run the race. Could it be accomplished even given my limitations? Could I train and run a marathon while eating three hundred calories a day?

Briefly, I begin to wonder what would occur if I did prescribe to this diet. I shudder to think of the consequences. What would result if I deliberately consumed these extra calories to aid my running? What would occur if I ate three-thousand calories one day and then it rained that same day? I'd be stuck inside with a belly full of disgusting food and no means by which to run off the calories. I'd be stuck inside feeling the fat pack take hold of my thighs. My jeans would get tighter. Tighter and tighter until the buttons popped off and the side seams split. I would gain back all that I've lost. I would lose that which I've already accomplished. I would weigh more than an elephant and thus be forced to run for five or six hours just to erase the calorie count.

There is no way I will follow such a diet. I don't even know why they presume to call it a diet when it seems like nothing more than a program for rapid weight gain.

I go back and read the chapter on distance intervals. Running four and five days a week, less than I do now, but running for longer periods. Could I do that? How? I'm taking twenty-one hours this semester plus rehearsing several nights a week. I barely have time to run the five miles even now. When would I fit in the time for the extra running? Would I even need to?

Then, I suddenly realize that the fall semester will be over at the beginning of December, and that our final performance will conclude on Christmas Eve. That gives me almost an entire month to work in the additional mileage needed.

I really want to try it. I want to know if I can run twenty-six miles. I want to see if I can run a marathon. If I can do this, perhaps there are other feats I can accomplish as well.

I won't tell anyone, though. I won't tell anyone of my plans. If I did, then I will have to live up to their expectations. I won't tell a soul. I will keep this my secret until I can determine whether or not it is possible.

November 5, 1984
Wt: 100 lbs.

During rehearsals, I gaze from my perch at the piano bench through the window panes into the surrounding avenue bungalows. I watch as the neighbors begin to gather onto their porches. It is as if our rehearsals prompt the automatic signal for them to leave the comfort of their central heat.

Despite the oncoming frost of the impending winter months, these neighbors resume their usual places upon their porch swings, wrapped in blankets while sipping wine and listening to the singing that comes from within our home.

A few have even thanked us for the live entertainment while others have asked that we open more windows so that they may better hear. Still others have told us that the music sparked an early longing for the Christmas spirit. These are the neighbors who already have their evergreens mounted and strung with lights in their living rooms.

I cannot recall the last time I've had this much fun or when I have laughed this hard. It has been since high school. The laughter has returned, the laughter that was hidden and ignored for too long. I am laughing again and it feels good. I am in my element behind the piano keys. Without knowing what the future holds, it feels that at this point in my life I am doing what I am supposed to be doing, in sync with the surrounding energy without knowing the outcome. I love the time that the four of us spend together in the bungalow each evening. I love being a part of a business that is fun, one I helped build from scratch.

I love that during this period of my life, the my music does not stay inside me, but rather has emerged and joined with that of these three friends.

I love that the response to our press kits was greater than originally anticipated.

I am not the least nervous about our performances, and that for me is a major milestone. Standing in front of others and performing would normally unnerve me. This time it does not for I am but one member of a group, and there is comfort in this. Armed with the comfort of the music that has never let me down, there is nothing to fear.

November 12, 1985
Wt: 101 lbs.

Figuring that if we don't sound good at least we'll look great, we splurge on forest green Victor Costa gowns. Helene insists that Christian Dior champagne hosiery is the only acceptable option to compliment the dresses. Another dozen bookings are added to the schedule. We are ready to perform.

With my great-aunt and uncle visiting from Shreveport, my mother asks if she can she bring them to a rehearsal. They will sit quietly, she says, and act as though they're not even present. She promises there will be no disruption from them. I ask the other girls for their blessing and am relieved by their eager response. Finally, a chance to test our material on a live audience.

November 13, 1985
Wt: 101 lbs.

My mother, aunt and uncle arrive early. Wearing a full-length mahogany mink coat, Aunt Netty looks as if she's dressed for the opera. My mother warmly greets my friends, happy to see them, and then begins to introduce her relatives who are not as interested in small talk as they are to listen to our progress. Without further intrusion, they take their seats on the Victorian couch where they remain respectfully silent, waiting.

Throughout the two-hour duration, they do not breathe a word as each melody is sung in four-part harmony. They make no attempts to clap between songs or excuse themselves for a bathroom break. But I can see they enjoy every minute of it. Their smiles give it away, the twinkles in their eyes. Aunt Netty has an arm around my mother, and Uncle Hugh holds Aunt Netty's free hand. They are smiling even though they don't realize it. As they sit sandwiched together, the elder trio seems lost in faraway memories of something good. I have had the Christmas spirit since early fall. Our neighbors have had it for months as well. Now my mother, aunt and uncle share it too.

They sit within the shadows of the living room lit only by a floor lamp propped next to the piano. Still, even in the dimness, their smiles glow through the shadows, smiles that remain glued, unmoved, unchanged. They are the guinea pigs, the measuring stick for whether or not we are ready for our first real performance. Until this point we were not certain. Their satisfied smiles now reveal the truth: *Yes, we are ready.*

November 15, 1985
Wt: 101 lbs.

My grandmother phones. Did I realize how upset my mother was after she left the rehearsal?

No, I did not have any sense that she was upset in the least, I tell her. In fact, I was under quite another impression.

"Well, apparently when they got back into the car, your Aunt Netty made some comment about how your legs looked like matchsticks, and that made your mother start crying. She was crying so hard she couldn't stop, so much that Uncle Hugh had to take her place at the driver's seat and drive everyone home. Aunt Netty didn't know what she could have possibly said to upset your mother like this, and your Uncle Hugh wanted to know why you were so thin – had you been ill? They said they'd never seen anyone so thin."

"What did Mom say?" I ask. I feel quiet, far away. I feel myself drifting far, far away.

"She didn't know what to say. She didn't know how to explain it. She didn't know how to explain why you've lost all that weight, why you're so thin."

I hang up the phone and feel terrible. I know my mother cried because of her worry. She is worried sick about me. I feel terrible because on the one hand I think I am getting better. I don't obsess over food every waking minute like I did this same time last year. And yet my weight has decreased even though this was not what I planned.

I don't obsess over food in the same way but perhaps that is because I don't need to. Perhaps it is because my body now knows instinctively the diet in which to adhere. Perhaps I don't obsess like I once did because I no longer feel hungry. The hunger pangs disappeared long ago. My mother is worried sick and I don't know what to do, how to change, how to comfort her, how to assure her that I am fine and that everything will be all right. I am happier here in the bungalow with my friends than I've been in years. I love this singing group, our first stab at entrepreneurship, the fact that I helped create something I love out of nothing. I feel better inside, and the gray clouds aren't as fierce and holding. I want her to know this. I don't want to hurt her. I want to pick up the phone and call her and tell her that I'm fine and to not worry.

But I don't call her. I don't phone to assure her that I'm fine. I am afraid this will only hurt her further. I do not want her to worry over me. I don't want her to spill any tears because of me. This is too much, too much. I want to call her and tell her all of this.

I dial and re-dial her number several times, but each time the phone rings I hang up. What is there to say? I cannot do it. I cannot convince her. I cannot convince myself.

December 13, 1985
Wt: 100 lbs.

We sang at the Reynolds' party, an evening soiree with more than two hundred guests dressed in tuxes, evening gowns and diamonds. There was a sumptuous buffet of eligible bachelors, many of whom asked for our telephone numbers. It was our best performance to-date. That is, until it ended.

Searching for Margaret, I walked into the kitchen where caterers and servers busily rushed about with Reed & Barton serving trays heaped with sturgeon and crab hors d'oeuvres and caviar, bringing in soiled linens and replacing the buffet with freshly ironed ones. When I couldn't find Margaret, I made my way into the living room where I walked smack into a gathered circle of five girls whom I was appalled to immediately recognize as those earlier tormentors from grade school. After all these years of no contact whatsoever, I found myself standing and staring face-to-face at the Mean Girls.

In the instant of recognition, I froze, stranded in time. The roar of the party silenced within my ears and I felt drawn back beneath the water, submerged in a floating state that was distanced from all reality. Christmas was suddenly nowhere to be found as the scent of holly, mistletoe and burning cherry candles seemed to disintegrate into the fading background. The aroma was instantly replaced by the once-familiar smell of those mothballs from the gray worn coat. In that moment, I had never progressed from the brick fortress of grade school. Nothing had changed, and life had not gone on. I felt like an idiot standing before them wearing my taffeta dress and champagne hosiery. They, too, seemed just as shocked to see me.

One by one they began to smile, not happy-to-see-you smiles, but the same jeering smirks I recognized from so long ago.

"Hey, Jackie," one said as casually as if I'd seen her just yesterday.

I felt their discerning gazes assess my attire, my hair, my skin, my overall appearance. And in that instant, my mind was immediately drawn back to the fretful, hopeless days of St. Ignatius. The old feelings were instantly relegated from the painful box of memories that I thought had been cast aside so long ago. Under their stares, I felt instantly microscopic, instantly worthless, and I began to inwardly cringe as all the memories began to flood back, all the name-calling, all the ridicule, all the jeers and back stabs. I was not worthy then, and even now, after all these years after the blissful parting, I feel the same sense of unworthiness return. It is back. Here it is. Yucky me. That little girl who was so despised assumes the place of the now-singer/college senior/businesswoman, and once again she is placed under the scrutiny of their merciless microscopic lens. Helpless, she cannot utter a word and she begins to stammer.

"I forgot something," I say, making a one-hundred-eighty-degree about-face, and then bound towards the front door exit.

Margaret reaches me just as I reach for the door handle and, upon taking one look at me and seeing my drawn ashen face, knows immediately that something is terribly, terribly wrong.

"What is it?" she whispers into my face. "What's wrong?" She says she's never seen me this upset.

"Nothing," I say, prying the door open and racing out onto the front porch, onto the sidewalk, towards my car. I cannot breathe. The air will not enter my lungs. I begin to see white spots before my eyes. My chest hurts. This dress feels too tight. I need to get out of here. Far away. As far away as the wind will take me.

I arrive home and spend two hours in the bathtub, scrubbing my skin over and over with a bar of Ivory. My roommate knocks repeatedly at the door.

"Are you all right," she asks.

I tell her I'm fine.

I barely speak for a week.

December 20, 1985
Wt: 99 lbs.

I wonder how different my life would be if I knew how to trust people more.

I imagine it to be more carefree like the lives of my siblings. I imagine it to be joyful and full of smiles, like the happy girls I see on television and read about in magazines.

I wonder what it would be like to trust people without having any fear that they will harm me, without automatically resorting to cynical thoughts of hidden agenda, that they are waiting for me to somehow expose myself in a negative manner, or that they await for me to make one slip so they can then stand back, point at me, and laugh.

It's not that I don't trust everyone. I have friends I would trust with my life and whom I feel would trust me with theirs. These are the friends from either high school, who somehow managed to put up with my habits, or my new friends, those I've made within the past two years well. I love all of these friends.

It is the outside world I do not trust, the outside world I fear, the outside world that spins on its axis, circling round and round in a definite rotation. All the world spins on the same axis. All the world except for mine that instead borders on the perimeter, watching and observing. Watching the earth spin and rotate, and wanting to jump onto that wide, blue map but somehow is unable out of fear.

Surely others must share at least some of these same issues. I know I wasn't the only girl taunted and ridiculed during my formative years. I know I wasn't the only girl hurt by a bad man. There were others. Many others. So why then do I feel like I am the only one? Is it because I live in a world where no one seems bothered by anything, where no one seems to have cares or concerns, where no one seems weighed down by the same darkness of the mind?

I want to be able to trust men without the fear that they will cause harm. Without fearing the same harm inflicted when I was a little girl.

The world does not want to see pain. It does not know how to deal with pain. The world wants to pretend that pain is no big deal and by doing so the world pretends that it can relieve the pain with an airy wave of a magical wand.

So why did it hurt me so deeply? Did I imagine the horror of those early years? Have I made too big a deal out of it, somehow relishing in the false security of being wounded? I don't want to be like that. I won't see myself as a victim, one who can never recover, or have others look upon me with pity.

Still, why does it continue to hurt?

December 25, 1985
Wt: 100 lbs.

Our singing season finale finally comes to a close. I received a gorgeous bouquet of yellow roses from Christopher, who is like my third brother, along with a note saying how much he enjoyed the music. The note is relegated to my special box of saved things.

December 26, 1985
Wt: 100 lbs.

I awaken from the most vivid dream I have ever had. It was so real that I question whether it was actually a dream at all.

It is the morning after Christmas. Fully dressed, I linger in my bedroom, putting away folded clothes in drawers, making my bed. I toss the emerald green Birds dress onto the farthest corner of the floor

*and remind myself to drop it off later at the dry cleaners. I am so
sick of wearing that dress night after night that I will not be sad
should it accidentally get lost at the cleaners.*

*I retrieve a paperback book from beneath my bed and then lounge
lazily atop the covers. There is no rush today. No appointments to
meet, no school, no more singing. This will be a lazy day. Perhaps
I will read until I fall asleep. A long afternoon nap followed by
more reading. Flipping through the novel's weathered pages, I locate
the dog-eared one where I last left off. I am alone in the bungalow,
alone in my room with the dancing blue flames of the space heater
to keep me warm.*

*Just then, the bedroom door suddenly swings open. Startled, I glance
to my right and there I see, standing in the threshold and smiling,
my piano teacher Miguel. His sudden apparition is as nonchalant
as if he saw me yesterday in his studio.*

*I am shocked by this sudden appearance that looks as human as
he did when he lived on earth. He wears the identical uniform
of clothing worn during all those years of lessons – black trousers
belted with a black leather belt and a long-sleeved sapphire-blue
collared shirt. Like before, the top button remains undone. A gold
pocket watch is concealed within his trousers pocket, and its long
gold chain dangles at his side. His smooth skin belies the eighty-two
years he lived on this plane, and his deep olive complexion remains
smooth and untouched. His white sparse hair is combed straight
back.*

*I cannot believe my eyes. I cannot believe this vision before me, and
yet I realize it is not a vision because of the woodsy fragrance of
his Old Spice cologne. My heart leaps and begins to beat faster
with happiness at seeing my old friend again. I can tell from his
expression that he is not angry with me for not having attended his
funeral. In fact, he seems just as happy as I am.*

I am so numb with shock that I cannot move, and I remain planted on my bed while witnessing this surreal happening before my very eyes. He takes a small step into the room and glances around at the bedroom furnishings, at the remaining few clothes strewn casually across the floor, at the tubes of makeup scattered atop the dresser. He smiles to himself, amused by what he sees. His nature was always gentle and this reflected in everything about him, from the way he spoke to the manner in which he dressed.

His hands are large as baseball mitts. I'd forgotten the singular caliber of those mighty hands that once swept across the piano keys, playing concertos by Mendelssohn, Liszt and Beethoven with the same ease as that of Twinkle Twinkle Little Star. I'd forgotten about those hands that once played at Carnegie Hall before relinquishing his concert status to return home and spend his remaining years teaching. How could I have forgotten those incredibly huge, capable hands? I had forgotten. Until now.

He takes another step, and then stops. Looking directly into my eyes, he begins to speak. "I came here to tell you something," he says with the faint traces of a Hispanic accent.

I still can't figure out if I'm dreaming or if this is a cruel vision created by the guilt and grief felt following his death. But the scent of his cologne wafts through the air, assuring me that this is real, that he really is here with me, right here and now, in this room at this point in time. I wonder what he has come to tell me, figuring that it must be fairly important to have travelled such a universal distance.

"I came to tell you I'm proud of you," he says matter-of-factly.

Tears begin to form and my heart begins to pound harder. I do not want to break down in front of him. I never did before and I will not now. Through his eyes, I was always seen as strong. He believed in me, and he believed in who I was. He saw me as a musician, and because of this, I learned to view myself in this same light. In his presence I always felt my strength because that was how he viewed me. How I love this man.

"I'm very proud of you," he repeats, staring at me with the intensity of an angel carrying implicit instructions. He then pauses as if waiting for a reply.

But I have no words apt for this unworldly communion. I cannot find anything suitable to say, and the familiar feelings of guilt begin to wash over me, guilt for having once disappointed him so. I don't deserve his kindness. I don't deserve the honor of his return. Oh if I could only take it all back, erase the past, told him I loved him, thanked him for what he did for me.

And yet I can tell by his actions, by his content countenance, that he harbors none of these negative feelings. There is no anger whatsoever in him. Only happiness. Only love. There is nothing to forgive. He already knows I love him. He wants me to let it go. He wants me to let it go. It is time to let these things go by the wayside. They have no place further in my life.

He remains standing unmoved from the same spot on the hardwoods. His black lace-ups shine against the oaken planks. Morning light floods through the open window blinds, shining into his eyes that do not blink.

"I'm proud of you and I'm going to tell you why," he continues. "You did something with your music. You did something good with it. You used your gift and created something with it, something wonderful. You shared it with others and gave them joy. And for that, I'm proud of you."

Then, before I have a chance to reply, he turns around and walks out of the room, closing the door behind him.

My eyes open and I glance at the rose wallpaper to my side, trying to figure out if I'm still lodged within this dream or if reality has set in. I don't recall dozing off, and feel disoriented. It didn't seem like a dream at all. It was as real as if Miguel were just here a second ago, standing here in this room and talking to me.

December 31, 1985
Wt: 102 lbs.

Ran three eight-mile stints this week. It's still a long way from twenty-six. Things have been quiet. No school. No work. Only running. Running and solitude.

I can hardly believe graduation is in May. What in the world am I going to do when I get out of school? I stand on the brink of being shoved out into the real world and have no clue where I'm going. I wish I could turn back the clock. I wish I could begin again as a freshman. I would take the pre-med biology and chemistry in order to know once and for all if I could pass these courses, to determine if medical school would have indeed been a possibility.

Is it possible to attain something that requires skills and abilities not innate to one's natural talents? Can't it be achieved by studying hard even with the assistance of a tutor if needed? Or are the natural gifts there for a reason? Like the piano, for instance. Because the gift was present, the assumption was that it was to be my life's purpose. And yet I knew this would never be the case. Guilt guilt guilt. Why is it assumed that a female is only capable of doing that which is immediately placed before her? If there is an interest in something other than an innate talent, then why is it so bad to want to pursue the other?

During high school, I spent many evenings in Mr. X's den where we would talk for hours. "Jackie, you are capable of accomplishing anything you want in this lifetime. Don't just assume that the predestined roles of a female are meant for you if you know in your heart this is not case, if you want to do something else."

He would talk to me, and encourage me to pursue my dreams. He urged me to think outside the box, and insisted that I believe my life had a definite purpose. I so wanted to believe him. I wanted to believe that I did have a purpose. He was the first to talk to me in this manner, to show me a world of possibilities that I had only dreamed of but didn't know existed. Our visits occurred during a time when the real world seemed so far away, years ahead when the unthinkable would occur: that I would live on my own, away from home. There didn't seem to be any rush at that time. After all, I had years to contemplate a future, and I was living in a happy time. I hadn't fallen off the cliff yet.

Yet here it is years after the fact, and I remember his words. I remember the care that he spent with me. I'm sure he has forgotten by now. But I haven't. Those words of his have suddenly reappeared and I remember as if it were yesterday. He planted seeds of hope, but I didn't realize it or fully appreciate it. Until now. Until now when I so desperately need to believe in *something*. When I need to believe in myself. There's no way either one of us could have known at that time just how much this would mean to me at this stage in my life when I do not know in which direction to turn.

Even after the mess I've created, his voice is still there, in the back of my mind, his voice, strong and assuring. "You can do anything you want. You can achieve anything you want in your life. You can make of your life what you want it to be."

Sometimes I read back through the journals I've kept since the age of thirteen. Curly-cued handwriting detailing the giddiness of a first crush, the humorous antics of high school, the intricacies of boyfriends, keg parties and prom nights, growing a marijuana plant in homeroom – a wild, overgrown, green thing that the teacher thought was the most beautiful topiary she'd ever seen, and notes concerning the all-important changing wardrobe.

I re-live the memories through the faded blue ink of a teenage girl's pen and, through tears of laughter and musings at the transitions from innocence, two things begin to dawn on me. The first is that I kept a written record at all. Without realizing it, I was transferring memories, thoughts and feelings from my heart and mind onto the pages of spiral notebooks. There has always been something within me that needed to write, something that required a pen in hand in order to satisfy a certain quench. There was something about writing that was uplifting and freeing. In this regard, I was the owl that spread its wings after the sun had long fallen, and soared above the earth in the night air, alone and free. My pen provided those wings.

The second discovery is that throughout the contents of dozens of journals, there remains a core issue that never wavers but, in fact, continues to reaffirm the older I got. It was the same issue at age thirteen as it was at the age of fifteen, and the identical issue at the age of eighteen as it is now at the age of twenty-one. It is a longing for independence. Financial independence, career independence. A longing to create something of my every own, unrelated to a husband or children. It is a unique identity and one that functions on its own.

Now, graduation looms around the bend, and I know that this is what I want: financial independence, a career. Yet I haven't a clue how to attain it, which career to pursue, which road to venture, how to form a plan. I haven't the foggiest notion what I should do and for that I feel like an utter failure. I want to be a success but I have not yet defined my interpretation of what this is.

When I ponder this predicament, it only makes me crazier. The anxiety worsens, making it impossible to think clearly about anything. The buzzing in my head continues, buzzing incessantly about nothing except for trying to look perfect, trying to maintain the perfect weight. I cannot think clearly about my future because this central thought – my weight – controls everything else. Going out into the world is so scary a thought that I feel I need to lose even more weight in order to be as perfect as I can be once I embark into that unknown abyss.

I feel so totally alone, and don't know how to find my path within this isolation. It is hard to reach out to others. The fear is always there – that they will judge me negatively, that I won't meet the expectation of others, and that I will fail. I don't know what to do. I don't know where to go.

January 10, 1986
Wt: 102 lbs.

The marathon is next week and I'm still not certain if I can run twenty-six miles. This week I ran a ten-mile and a thirteen-mile. I don't think I can make it much further than thirteen miles. Still, perhaps I should try anyway. However, I would hate to try and then be able to only run half the distance. Failure!

I shouldn't even be focusing on the marathon. I should be concerned with plans after graduation. If only I had a crystal ball to help me figure out in which direction to go. Why is this so difficult?

January 19, 1986
Wt: 102 lbs.

Finished the race in four hours, fifty-six minutes.

What a charge the day was. I've never experienced anything like it. It began in the early morning of a chilly downtown. There were thousands of runners. I had no idea there were so many runners in the city. There were the serious runners, those whose muscles ripple throughout every inch of their thighs, calves, biceps, and triceps. And then there were the beginners and the intermediates, all wearing the prestige of an assigned number pinned to the backs of their t-shirts. Even before the race began there was a charge in the air, an excitement as everyone kept in motion in attempt to abate exposure from the cold.

Then the starting gun sounded and the pack of runners slowly began to move forward. Crowds filled the surrounding sidewalks and curbs, waving signs and offering orange slices. Crowds cheered and waved banners and signs for those whom they knew in the race. Their cheers and whistles were met with the sounds of thousands of pairs of tennis shoes plodding against the asphalt, all galloping down Main Street.

Running with the pack, I felt a part of something big. Something so large that even with the diversity in backgrounds, each shared a common purpose and goal: to complete the race.

I still don't know how I made it to the eighteenth mile but somehow my blistered feet kept moving forward, making steady progress. I am ready to quit right then and there, and am just about ready to call it quits when I look up and see my sister Leslie. She has apparently been standing by in the curb with the rest of the crowd for quite some time. She is wearing a new running outfit. We spot each other at the same time and our eyes lock. I slowly make my way to her side. I am ready to go home. I want to quit. I am exhausted and my feet are blistered.

Immediately recognizing the fatigue, her grin grows even broader and she nudges me back into the middle of the street. Her arm presses against my back as she maneuvers me in and out of the throngs of runners to an empty space on the pavement that is then replaced with the two of us. My sister begins to run at my side. She pats my back and says she is not about to let me quit. She says she has come to run the last eight miles with me. She knew this final leg is the most difficult stretch of the course, and therefore she will not allow me to come this far only to quit now. She promises that we will finish together.

A few more miles down the road, the fatigue began to worsen and I have no idea how I will ever finish. I cannot go any further. My legs are steel blocks, numb and aching. I want a Snickers bar. I want some Mexican food. I want to put my feet up. I want to soak my limbs in a salty bath. But Leslie is not about to let me quit. She says *Just get that far*, and then points to some innocuous landmark, another baby step on which to focus, a block farther up the road. Then once we meet that destination, she points to another landmark and prods me to go a little further.

It is after another mile when I happen to gaze into the crowd and to my surprise see none other than Ronald and Nancy Reagan – Margaret and Helene wearing their Halloween masks from the previous October. Ronnie wears a brown raincoat and flashes peace signs with her fingers to the oncoming runners who are amused that president of the United States has come out to witness this event. Another mile down the road we happen across Teddy who also has been apparently waiting in the sidelines for some time. Once he sees me and my sister, he cheers and claps and encourages us to keep moving forward. We do not stop to talk. If we did, it would be impossible to pick up again. We wave hello and keep going, and inwardly I feel happy at the support of my friends. In fact, I know they have been showing their support all along, through everything. But I have been mostly oblivious to this.

My sister continues to say *you can do it. You can do it.* She continues to point to landmarks as baby-step destinations which we reach together. She does this for the last remaining miles, all the way until the two of us finally cross beneath the waving red flag of the finish line.

After returning home, I receive a phone call from a neighbor. She congratulates me and says, "If you can run a marathon, you can accomplish anything you want with your life. Nothing is impossible for you. I want you to remember this – that you did something that you did not believe was possible. All things are possible for you."

February 16, 1986
Wt: 103 lbs.

I enroll in a marketing class with the assumption that it will be an easy A.

How wrong I was. In fact, it has been the most difficult class of my college career. The workload is tremendous, not at all what I assumed. But what becomes quickly apparent is the fact that this instructor is a stickler for good writing.

"In this world, the ability to write well is as important as the ability to speak well," he says. He believes these two items are the keys to opening doors of many opportunities.

My papers are returned to me with his furious scribbling in red ink that take up every inch of space within the margins. He suggests sentence re-structures, more precise wording and correct use of grammar. Yet despite the rest of the class's bemoaning this perceived harsh criticism on their papers as well, ("this isn't an English class!"), I am secretly thrilled. I can learn much from him. Through what seems an accidental coincidence of fate, I can learn to become a better writer. This teacher, who is not aware of my evening writing rituals or the dozens of journals stored under lock and key, will show me how to improve this skill. I view it as a blessed opportunity, a challenge. He will never know how much this means to me. I will not tell him because if I do, my fear is that I will then have to live up to a new set of expectations on his part. No, I will keep it to myself. I will take all of his written remarks to heart, learn from them and thus hone that which I have always done.

March 9, 1986
Wt: 101 lbs.

Two months until graduation. I can no longer hide from this dreaded date or pretend that this next major phase of my life is about to begin. I wish it was not so near, teasing and taunting the fact that I remain clueless as to what to do. I am so petrified about this transition that all I think about is food. Food that never enters my mouth. The few calories a day that are immediately jogged away so that no weight will accumulate on this body. I cannot control anything. Not the graduation that looms right around the corner or the emptiness inside that provides no compass to direct my path. All of my friends know exactly what their plan is. I am the only one left in the dark.

March 15, 1986
Wt:

Dr. Hops asks me to stay after class. I don't know why. "Come with me up to my office," he says, removing his eyeglasses and placing them in his shirt pocket.

I follow him up the linoleum stairs. Black wrought-iron handrails are icy to the touch. Everything seems cold. I am always cold. Even with the oncoming heat of Houston, my fingers and toes remain cold all the time.

The upper staff offices are deserted as he leads me to his. A swift gaze discerns that his neat office matches the persona he exudes. Papers and files are set in neat piles upon the desktop. A few framed photographs set within an otherwise empty bookcase. He takes a seat behind the desk and I sit in the empty chair in front.

"I'm worried about you," he says earnestly.

"Me?" I have been absent from numerous classes. Still, I don't know why he would particularly care as there is nothing that makes me stand out in class.

"You've missed four classes in the past two weeks. That's not like you."

I feel embarrassed. Lately I've felt so drained that all I want to do is sleep. The need for sleep is so strong that I have taken to napping and thereby missed the afternoon teachings. The daily naps offer no relief as I do not ever awaken feeling refreshed. Rather, I awaken with the same ongoing sense of dread. Fear is the first thing I feel when I awaken. Fear stays with me throughout the day, and never leaves.

"Are you okay?" he asks.

I pull my pink sweater tighter around my shoulders. I am so cold in here. I wish someone would turn off the air-conditioner. I look at the thermostat on the wall and see that it is already turned off.

"I'm fine." The words are barely a whisper. Everything feels so dark and isolated.

His earnest expression is not willing accept this excuse so lightly. "You just seem so tired. You always look like you're about to fall asleep in class."

"I haven't been sleeping well," I say. "I've been tired lately and have fallen asleep in the afternoons. I didn't wake up in time to get here. I'm sorry."

"I'm not worried about the missed classes," he says. "I'm worried about you. You have become even thinner than when this class first began at the beginning of the semester. I'm really worried." He taps a pencil on his desk. "Do you think perhaps you need to go to a doctor?"

"I guess I'm just a little stressed out is all," I say. "Really, I'm fine. I just needed some rest." I want to sleep for forever.

"What's causing the stress?" he asks.

"Oh, everything and anything," I reply. "Graduation is right around the corner and I don't know what to do." I am surprised at my honesty as I know I am exposing a major weakness. The weakness of being so clueless.

"I see," he says. "You're worried about finding a job."

"I'm worried about trying to figure out what to do," I say.

"Perhaps you're approaching this the wrong way," he says. "Perhaps you're viewing this as so many others do – by placing yourself in the passive position of taking whatever is offered."

I nod. It is true although I despise the notion that I could be so passive. I despise passivity. Not taking charge. Not taking action. Not doing anything. Yet, isn't this exactly what I've done?

He continues. "Perhaps you need to take some time to ponder exactly what it is that you want to do."

"I don't think there is anything for me," I say.

"Sure there is," he says, pointing to his brain and then to his heart. "It is there, within you. You just haven't tapped into it yet."

I do not know why I am telling him this. I don't know what sudden urge has come over me to allow myself to expose such weakness. But for some reason, I do not feel he is judging me as I so often fear. He is only trying to help, and this time I will take the help.

He continues. "Is there anything right off the top of your head – something you can see yourself doing?" he asks.

I shake my head.

"What about your music? Any career there?"

I shake my head again. "Definitely not. I don't want to be a piano teacher."

He nods. "I understand. I agree, I think you're cut out to do something else. What other interests are there?"

I tell him that business interests me. I tell him about the music ensemble and just how much I enjoyed creating a profitable business. I also tell him of my fascination with economics even though I haven't figured out how to apply this to a career in business. Then I add, "I like to write as well."

He leans back in his chair, looks up into the ceiling, and ponders. Then he speaks again.

"You see? You think you have no interests, that you will not be good at anything. But do you realize quite the opposite is true? That, in fact, you have many interests. Plus a true love of writing. Believe me, there is a place for you out in the world. Somewhere that will combine all of these things."

"But where?" I ask.

"My dear, you are going to have to find that out for yourself."

"How? I don't know how." Why can't somebody just give me the answers?

"By taking some time to ask yourself these questions: What is it I truly want to do? What career is it that I want? You need to place yourself on the opposite side of the fence – the side that places *you* in control of your destiny. Believe me, once you ask these questions, the answers have a mysterious way of returning to you."

"It sounds too easy," I say.

"Discovering yourself is the easy part," he replies. "Accepting yourself is usually what is so often difficult."

April 20, 1986
Wt: 100 lbs.

I lack nine credit hours to graduate in May. When the guidance counselor delivers this unexpected news, I freak. I begin to cry. I bawl. It is an outburst like no other in years as I feel the whole world slipping further beyond my control. How could I have been so stupid to have not realized this before? How could I have allowed this to surprise me so unexpectedly? The guidance counselor says it is because of my having transferred schools.

I realize that my college time is over. I had four years to get in and out of school. Four years and not a day longer because my brothers and sisters are standing in line behind me, waiting for their turn. My parents are spending every penny earned on our education and now I have gone and blown it.

However, my mother doesn't seem to mind the news at all. Nor does she seem the least bit bothered when I tell her of an off-campus Spanish curriculum in Mexico that would fulfill these last needed credits. The class starts in June and I'll be finished by the mid-July. A college graduate.

My mother says that my fluency in Spanish will help facilitate the course. She urges me to go. She says I can use the extra time to figure out a plan for myself. She says there is something about getting away from one's surroundings that frees the mind and allows all creativity to enter. She says perhaps this is a blessing in disguise. She tells me not to worry about the money. The more she considers the program, the more she views it as a wonderful opportunity.

You go and get some rest there," she says. "Get away from here and soak in the warm beaches of the Atlantic. See if that doesn't help to discover a fresh new mindset. It will bring about rejuvenation, healing, and then you'll then know better what your next step is."

I feel better after talking to her. Perhaps this really isn't the worst thing that could ever happen to me. I can definitely use the extra time.

Just as my instructor suggested, I have mentally posed the question: *What do I want to do?* I have placed the mental energy out there, into that unseen realm that supposedly gathers all information and returns with the gifts of knowledge and awareness. He insisted that many answers are received in this manner, and that patience is a must in the interim until the answers arrive. I am still waiting for a response.

June 5, 1986
Wt: 102 lbs.

Don knows what he wants. He has never allowed his immigration from Eastern Europe to hinder any of his goals. Despite the struggle of having to learn English as a teenager, he has always managed to always stay at the top of his class. After graduation, he plans to attend Harvard Law School on a full scholarship. He says that while he does not yet know exactly how this will be accomplished, somehow he intuitively knows the dream will indeed materialize. He is committed to making this happen.

Knowing that I leave tomorrow for Merida, he arrives at the bungalow bearing a gift, a tiny bundle wrapped neatly within a brown paper sack. Despite its small size, it is much heavier than it appears. I unfold the tight creases and peer inside. "This is something that helped to change my life," he says while I remove the thickest paperback book I've ever seen, and glance at the unfamiliar cover and author's name. It is titled 'Atlas Shrugged.'

"Take this book with you and read it while you're away," he urges. "I think it will help you just as it did for me."

I leaf through the contents and discover it contains more than a thousand pages. He says it is not a book that can be read in a week, but rather over a longer period and requires much deliberation in-between. There is much insight contained within, he says, and the south-of-the-border sojourn allows for the ideal time to read and contemplate. He believes that it will help me in more ways than I can imagine.

After he leaves, I sit quietly on the front porch swing. The book rests in my lap, unopened. Sprinkles of kindness have surrounded me always, even during these past years when I felt totally alone. I begin to realize just how many people have tried to help me. Most through small, unexpected ways. I begin to realize that throughout this self-imposed exile and imprisonment of denials, that I was never truly alone and that many others were watching, waiting for the right moment to intervene when they could offer any assistance whatsoever. Even this book – a gift of the heart from someone who truly doesn't have a dime – is yet another sign that I am not alone, and that others care. This person scraped together money he didn't have because he cared. I have lived in a world of self-isolation, but I am just beginning to realize that I was never truly alone.

July 16, 1986
Wt: 102 lbs.

This past month has been a blessing in which to focus and re-think my future. I recall little of the time spent in Spanish classes or the hours pored over homework assignments. Even the mellow breezes of the Atlantic and the spicy smell of baking tamales at corner restaurants are secondary to this all-consuming passion of reading the book.

It never leaves my hands, my eyesight, my thoughts during any time not reserved for those related to class. Hours spent in isolation either curled up on my top bunk or relaxing in a lawn chair with the Yucatan gulf spread before me provide the calm setting for the reading of this book that has provided a much-needed focus. It took the full six weeks to complete, during which I constantly marveled at the fact that my friend provided me with the precise tool needed at this point in my life.

Now I know what I want to do. Finally, there is a direction.

July 17, 1986
Wt: 103 lbs.

I want to work for an advertising agency. I figure that will combine both the business interests and the writing skills within a creative environment. I do not have any pre-conceived notion of the outcome over the next several years. But for now, it is the place to start.

The city's economy is not doing well, and most of the Savings & Loans have declared bankruptcy. As a result, there is a glut of homes for sale with little demand to alleviate this once-booming real estate market. The stock market continues to decline as well. Headlines from the Business section profile all the companies that are having to lay off employees. Needless to say, it is not the most opportune market for a recent college grad with no experience. But somehow, I will figure out a way to make it work. Somehow I will land a job in advertising.

July 20, 1986
Wt: 103 lbs.

Once again I entertain the familiar wooden hallways of the Rice library. Many hours of research unearth a lengthy list of advertising firms located here in town. They are of all shapes and sizes, different strengths within different industries. But of all the firms I read about, one company stands out above the rest. It is not only the largest, but has been in business the longest as well. Its client roster includes chain restaurants, car dealerships, nonprofit organizations, law firms and medical facilities, real estate companies. They seem to handle all types of works and understand numerous types of industries. There would be much to learn at a company like this. Much for me to learn. I want to work for this company. This company and no other. This is where I want to start. This is where my future will begin. Somehow I will get my foot in the door.

August 5, 1986
Wt: 103 lbs.

The Human Resources Director tells me there are no openings. He says that due to the city's business decline, the agency has had to lay off thirty employees within the past month. He explains that the first expense that most companies cut when faced with a belt-tightening is the ad budget. The agency has already lost many key people and is in desperate need of new business in order to stay afloat. He says there are no open positions and wishes me luck in my job search.

I do not want to leave. I want to work here. Nowhere else but here. My gut tells me this is where I need to be. This is where I will start.

Surely there is at least one position, I say. He scans my resume. Good grades and a member of the honor society combined with the illustrious past positions of waitress, lifeguard, sales clerk and the Christmas quartet. They don't hire fresh out of college, he says. Experience is required.

I tell him that this is the only company I want to work for. I explain that my mind was already made up even before any interviews were set based upon my research. I explain my reasons for wanting to work here.

A quizzical expression crosses his face. It seems he does not know quite what to make of me. He peruses the scant resume once again.

Well, he says, there is one opening. But only one. But he doesn't feel I would have any interest in it. He says I am overqualified, and I try not to laugh out loud, knowing full well I am not overqualified for anything.

What is it? I ask.

Administrative assistant to the director of public relations, he says. The salary is very low.

I cannot believe my luck, realizing that public relations involves extensive writing skills. I would learn so much and this would only open more doors.

When can I start? I ask.

August 30, 1986
Wt: 103 lbs.

Janice, my new boss, is almost apologetic every time she asks me to type her materials. It's as if she feels the need to go out of her way to make me not feel like the lowest man on the totem pole. I am grateful for her sense of decency, and tell her honestly that I do not mind in the least. I do not mind the grub chores because every letter that is typed, every press release, every report, every new business presentation, ever campaign offers more opportunities to learn.

I do not merely type and return the materials but rather, take the time to study her unique writing style, the various uses of a hard vs. a soft lead, the personification of words that assume an easy conversational tone. I study the format of each press release and how a huge compilation of research is developed into a new business pitch. There is much to learn and I will learn it all. And in the meantime I am also learning about many different types of industries.

She is amused when I ask for permission to take older files home with me. What for? she asks. To study, I explain. I want to learn to write like you, I say.

She nods, chuckling, and asks that I return them when I'm finished.

September 15, 1986
Wt: 103 lbs.

A small poster tacked onto a bulletin board in the coffee room catches my eye. It is a photograph of a young local attorney in dire need of a liver transplant. Because of the operation's large expense, the family has instigated a city-wide plea for help.

Removing the poster, I carry it to Janice's office and set it on her desk where she is studiously bent over a pile of work.

"Not now," she says, dismissing me in an offhand gesture.

"This will just take a second," I say.

Pointing to the smiling black and white portrait, I say, "This young man needs some help."

"So send him a check," Janice says.

"No," I say. "We will help him."

Janice stares at my bald audacity. "And how do you propose we do so?"

"If he's an attorney that means he's a member of the local bar association," I reason.

"So?" Janice says. But she is listening.

"I've seen the mailing list for the P.R. materials we sent to all the members of the state Trial Lawyers Association. There are thousands on that list. Which means there are many on the list for the local association. We could hold a fundraiser. An after-work cocktail hour held at one of the restaurants we have on our client roster. I don't feel the restaurant would turn us down because it should bring in a ton of revenue from the alcohol alone. We will send a letter to each member of the local Bar Association explaining this cause, and invite them to come make a donation."

"What if, instead, we just ask for a specific amount?" she asks.

"No," I reason. "These attorneys have big pockets. This is a generous city, even with the economy in the toilet. We will simply suggest that they bring their checkbooks."

Janice sits back in his chair and ponders the possibility. "Yes," she says, "I believe that would work. Thing is, though, I don't have enough time to fit another project into my schedule. Perhaps we could put this on the back burner for a few months until some of the other projects clear."

"No," I say. "He needs this operation now. I'll take care of all the details."

September 26, 1986
Wt: 103 lbs.

Dad calls unexpectedly and invites me to lunch.

We meet at a swanky Italian restaurant where starched white linens and fresh roses add to the ambience of a resplendent interior. Dad looks good, and tells me that he is doing well. We chit-chat and I enjoy this time alone with my father. Having not seen him in several weeks, I miss him. We order quickly.

"How's the job going?" he asks.

"Great," I reply. "I love it." I explain the various tasks I've been assigned and what I am learning. I tell him how great my new boss is.

My father nods and smiles as he listens attentively. He fiddles with his gold cufflinks, his favorites, the ones with the embossed tigers. When I was little, I thought they represented an earlier job pumping gas at the filling station.

After the waiter sets our plates in front of us, my father says, "There's something I want to talk to you about. Something your mother and I have discussed."

"Shoot," I say.

"We're really proud of you getting this job and all," he begins, "and we know you'll do well. But we're still worried about your weight. You're still not eating. We know this remains a problem for you, and we want to help. We want you to consider going to a treatment center."

I am utterly shocked by this request, stunned that my parents have still not let go of the issue. And yet, I realize it is only because of their love for me.

"I think I am getting better," I say, although the reality is that not an ounce has been gained. "Mentally," I say, "I feel there have been some changes although I can't really explain it. But for the first time it feels as if I'm moving forward. And with a purpose."

My father listens and nods. The disappointment is evident in his expression. "I'm really glad to hear that," he says, "but that doesn't hide the fact that the issue still remains. All your mother and I care about is that you are healthy and happy. The not-eating has gone on now for several years. It's a miracle you're even alive. We want to help keep you alive. Can you understand that?"

"Yes," I say, meaning it.

I think back to my youth and all the years of my father coming home from work after helping families deal with their loved ones' deaths. His is not just a job but rather, a calling, one in which I've always felt that only a few are called because of the emotional stress. My father not only possessed the strength but he was superior at what he did. I know this because others told me. Others whom he helped.

However, despite his unwavering strength, there was one issue that never failed to crush his strength. And that was when he dealt with a family that had lost a child. For those, the most difficult of funerals, he remained strong and courageous throughout the preparations, wake, church service and gravesite burial. He remained a rock, the backbone while parents poured out their grieving hearts to him as they dealt with the unthinkable task of burying their child. Dad remained strong until the minute he walked through the door at home. At that point, he slipped off his shoes at the door and, in stocking feet, walked straight to the Lazy-Boy in the den where he plopped his worn-out self upon the cushion and sobbed for hours. It was on these rare evenings when he never failed to tell each of us kids, individually, how much he loved us, how he would do anything for us, how he would never survive should something like that happen to one of us.

Now, sitting beside him, I know too well the emotional hardship I have imposed upon both him and my mother. I am fully aware of how difficult this is for him. I fully realize what has been going on in his mind, the dread of not wanting to lose his child. I despise myself for hurting him so, for causing this pain. Perhaps, I think to myself, perhaps I could attend a weekend session, something that would not require much time. I do not have much free time as it is.

"How long is the treatment?" I ask.

"Forty-five days," he says. He tells me about two centers, one in Houston, the other in Dallas. I can choose which one.

I shake my head at the length of time, knowing it is out of the question. "But what about work?" I say. "I just started.

I can't take time off now. They'll fire me. I can't just up and leave for forty-five days."

"I know that," he says. "Your mother and I have discussed that as well. And we're prepared to help you for as long as it takes to get you back on your feet should you decide to go and your employers then choose to replace you. We'll support you for however long it takes."

Even if I agree, I know my parents do not have the extra money to pay for the exorbitant cost of treatment. And now Abigail is in college. Three kids in college at the same time. Just as it has been for years. My going to a treatment center would only add to their already difficult hardship. They love me. My actions have set terror in their hearts and they are willing to do anything it takes to see me well. I hate the fact that I have caused them this pain. I love them and do not want to hurt them further.

But this is one request I cannot grant. For once, the earth begins to feel solid underneath my feet. To leave my job now would surely bring back the blacker, bleaker feelings of yesterday, and add to the anxiety of having to start all over again. The vicious cycle would only worsen.

"Dad," I say as gently as I know how. "I appreciate you. I really do. I appreciate everything you and Mom have tried to do for me. I am so sorry for all this pain I have caused you." I want to be able to explain everything to him, to explain the reasons why I do not eat and why I continue to run even though my clothes are practically falling off. I want him to know that I am not trying to hurt him, and that I know I am hurting myself. But I do not know how to explain because I don't even understand. I don't know why this all started in the first place, or why I can't get the cycle to stop.

He looks down, as if he has already guessed my answer.

"But I can't," I continue, staring into his eyes, pleading. "I cannot leave at this point. I cannot just throw away what I've accomplished. I just can't."

Even I realize I have not accomplished very much. Not really. But at least, for me, it is something. Something from which to build. A direction in which to head.

Despite everything, he doesn't appear too shocked. Although I know he'd hoped for a different outcome, he doesn't appear surprised by the final verdict. His big blue eyes wander off into the distance beyond the window's view, and now he is the one who seems very far away. He knows he is the one who now has to go home and deliver the news to my mother. He wishes he could tell her something different.

He says, "Jackie, should you ever change your mind, the offer will always be open."

"I know," I say.

October 16, 1986
Wt: 102 lbs.

To everyone's surprise, the restaurant had barely enough room to accommodate all the attorneys who turned out for the benefit. The manager, thrilled by the non-stop ringing of the cash register, agrees to donate a portion of the bar proceeds to our cause.

Janice and I sit at a front table where we accept the donations, an outpouring of generosity I did not expect, the magnanimous pouring-out of cash by hundreds of attorneys present to help one of their own. The affair, set to end at 7:30 p.m., was still going strong after nine o'clock. Finally, after eleven p.m., we head for the manager's back office to tally the money. We count and then, not believing the final sum, re-count. We do this several more times because we can't believe it is true. In our hands, in stacks of checks and green paper bills, we are holding more than thirty-five-thousand dollars, more than enough to pay for the operation.

October 20, 1986
Wt: 103 lbs.

The girls want to revive our music quartet for the upcoming holiday season. Christmas is right around the corner. With everyone's time constraints and full-time jobs, there is now less time for rehearsals than last year. Nonetheless, the gig is on. We are back in business.

October 25, 1986
Wt: 102 lbs.

Janice includes me in client meetings and project-planning sessions. At this early career stage, I have nothing to offer, no pearls of wisdom to share with these business executives. She wants me to just sit back, listen and learn. I learn much. I watch and observe how she deals with clients, with the same ease as that of old friendships. Her manner is easy and comfortable and in this respect she reminds me of my brothers and sisters, and of my father.

She gives me one opportunity after another to learn the trade from her long distinguished career. And in return, she asks very little. One thing she does ask for is my company with her and the rest of the department when they go to lunch. She asks this on a regular basis. But I do not oblige. I never say yes. It is the same old pattern, the same mindset of not wanting to expose my eating habits. I do not want them to watch as I eat a plain salad void of any real nutrition. I do not want them to start asking questions. I do not want to confirm their suspicions. I do not want them to pry. I do not want to be judged. Especially now. Especially when I've worked so hard and want to keep learning more, progressing forward. I do not want their interpretation of my eating habits to potentially prohibit any opportunities I might have here.

I know I can overcome this. Somehow. There has got to be a way. I'm just not sure what it is though. I love my work here and that in itself is a major feat. At least for me. I know I can do better, learn more, rise within the ranks of this company, acquire so many useful skills that other companies will want to hire me. For the first time I see the opportunities. I see the potential. I must continue to move forward.

While I don't care so much what the other members of our small P.R. group think, I do care what my boss thinks. In fact, I care a great deal because she has taught me so much and shown a great deal of kindness. Because of this, I do not want to disappoint her by somehow exposing my weakness, the weakness of not eating properly. Janice has never once harped on me about my weight. She never says 'Eat something! Eat a sandwich!" like the others occasionally do.

I happen to glance through the glass window pane into the lush tropical gardens of the courtyard, and see Janice taking a rare afternoon break on a park bench. I walk outside and sit beside her. The sun beats overhead, and the faint roar of the nearby freeway is the only sound to enter this green haven of park benches. Out of the blue, she tells me of her concern for her grown daughter. I didn't even know she had a daughter. She says her daughter is very thin, and she suspects the girl does not eat properly. She wonders aloud if there is an eating-disorder issue going on.

My sense is that this is not attempt to pry into my life or my personal issues. My sense is that she feels there may be a problem, and that perhaps in some odd, related way I might provide some clue or answer. My sense is that she has not discussed this too much, with family or anyone. My sense is that she has no more of the answers than any of us do.

She says she doesn't know what to do, how to approach her daughter, or if she even should. She worries all the time.

I tell her that my parents, too, worry about the same thing. I tell her that I don't know how my life got this way, but that even without personally knowing her daughter, that I am certain of one thing – this girl needs her unconditional love.

October 31, 1986
Wt: 104 lbs.

Amidst the hoopla of the entire agency costumed for Halloween, there is yet another larger underlying excitement. Apparently, the owner's son has resigned his executive position at a top Los Angeles agency to return home and now work at his father's side. The whispers began a week ago.

What does this mean? Will there be a re-structure? Will there be favoritism? Always the whispering, nervous wonderings over what this means. I cannot help but overhear the chatter that gathers in the hallways and coffee room as his impending arrival nears.

His arrival means nothing to me for I am focused on learning mode. My daytime job, coupled with evenings rehearsals leave little time to think of much else.

Janice calls a meeting with the tiny public relations group. She is tired of hearing the same incessant chatter and wants it to stop. She says, "We will treat him with the same respect we give to any new employee."

On the day of his arrival, I go out of my way to avoid him. After all, he *is* cute, and I don't want to meet someone for the first time wearing the ridiculous costume of 'two heads are better than one', a Styrofoam model's head complete with makeup and blonde wig affixed to my left shoulder.

November 5, 1986
Wt: 104 lbs.

The minute I get home the phone rings. I do not know how he got my number. I have barely said two words to him since he started at the agency. He jokes and says his feelings are hurt that I left the office without saying goodbye. I am not amused. I ask if he feels there is a stigma attached to being the boss's son. He says he expected it so it doesn't bother him although he does admit it feels a little strange calling his father by his first name. Thus begins a conversation that lasts nearly four hours.

He wants to take me out this Saturday. Nope, I say. Too much to do. Full schedule. It is a lie that I try to disguise well because I don't want to hurt his feelings. He seems a good-enough guy. And if it weren't for the fact that he was the owner's flesh and blood I would definitely be up for the date. However, for now I don't want to get tangled up in any office politics. I don't want to do anything that could potentially threaten my job.

November 10, 1986
Wt: 104 lbs.

The man is definitely persistent. He won't take no for an answer despite my repeated excuses. I realize that he is not going to walk away so easily, and even though his interest is flattering, my mind is made up. Going out with him would be disastrous. Surely nothing good would come out of it. And then I would have the stigma of dating the boss's son. I would be viewed as nothing more than giddy chattel rather than the serious nature I try to portray. If I venture out on a date with him and this was discovered by my co-workers, no one at the office would ever take me serious again.

November 11, 1986
Wt: 104 lbs.

I ask my mother what to do. I explain the situation, explain about the evening phone calls, and how I have consistently refused his every attempt to take me out. I have run out of excuses.

My mother asks if he is cute.

Yes, I admit. He's the most handsome man I've ever met.

She wants to know if he is smart.

Yes, I admit again. He's a natural speaker, quick-thinking on his feet, a whiz at his job. Particularly interested in American history and politics. He's an avid reader too and I think he's read as many novels as I have. In fact, there's hardly a topic he can't discuss with a great depth of knowledge and understanding. He has a great sense of humor and a sharp wit as well. He makes me laugh. He is a good listener. And even though our friendship thus far is confined mainly to phone conversations, already there is an equality and a matching of minds that I have never before experienced. As I continue to verbally cite the long list of his many attributes, it is as if I too am hearing the fullness and uniqueness of him for the first time. It begins to dawn on me that I have standing right here before me the ideal man.

My mother verbalizes my exact thoughts. She says she doesn't see what the problem is.

I explain the office politics dilemma, the potential repercussions from dating the boss's son.

But what harm can come of a single date, she says.

If the date goes sour, I say, so does my career.

Oh, she says.

I say that he's just asking me out because he's trying to re-build his life again in his hometown. Perhaps he's just lonely. I know plenty of women who would love to go out with him. In fact, the entire agency is filled with women, more than half of whom are single. This is certainly not a man who need struggle for a date. Not with his looks and charm. I have plenty of friends who would love to go out with him.

An idea begins to form in mind while I assume the role of matchmaker. Yes, that's it. This is too perfect. I will fix him up with one of my friends. He will be happy and my friend will be thrilled. He will like her so much that his energy and time will thus be transferred elsewhere. It will then be out of my hands and I can resume my concentration on my job and the singing group. Yes, what a good idea. So perfect that I can't believe I hadn't thought of it before. By this weekend he will have a date. It just won't be me.

November 23, 1986
Wt: 103 lbs.

He is not amused by my attempt to play matchmaker.

I show him a glossy 8 x 10 portrait of Kristen and explain that she works as model. Translation: beauty. He looks at it as uninterested as if it were a bologna sandwich. I am amazed by his lack of enthusiasm as everyone else who views the photograph shows instant interest in meeting the mysterious woman behind the Ultra-Brite smile.

I tell him that not only is she single but also she happens to be available this upcoming Saturday night.

He turns back to the pile of work on his desk and says he is busy, that we will discuss it another time.

I walk out of his office feeling somewhat relieved even though it's not a match — yet. I am relieved but at the same time a little sad as I have come to look forward to his phone calls. I enjoy our conversations. I am strongly attracted to him. The more I get to know him, the more I want to know. However, this is probably just one of those instances of being in the wrong place at the wrong time.

November 24, 1986
Wt: 104 lbs.

This time he calls before eight a.m. I am just about to leave for work when the phone rings.

"Look," he says. "I don't want to go out with any of your friends although I'm sure they are quite lovely. I want to go out with *you*. This weekend is my birthday and the only thing I want for my birthday is to spend an evening with you. So what do you say?"

I am more flattered than I have ever been in my life. I do want to go out with him. I have been denying that truth just as much as I have denied myself food all these years. And besides, how could I ever dismiss his risk at appearing a fool by revealing such raw honesty.

I look at the calendar. It will be Thanksgiving weekend and the first of our singing performances begin this Friday night. Saturday day and evening are also booked solid. I tell him this. I say that I don't expect to get home until after midnight on Saturday.

"Okay, then," he says. I hear him smile. "I'll pick you up at half past midnight."

December 20, 1986
Wt: 104 lbs.

As long as I live, I will never forget what happened at tonight's performance.

There is no feeling to compare with the satisfaction and peace from providing Christmas spirit through music to others or looking out into a crowd and watching their expressions change upon hearing a favorite holiday tune. I am a silent witness to long-ago memories that are instantly relegated, colors and music from a time of yesteryear as the quartet sings one song after another. Each performance has its own unique and satisfying quality. But none of this can compare to the miracle I witnessed tonight.

The Steinway grand graces the center of Neiman Marcus. The store has been professionally decorated – weeks spent adorning the glass escalators, shelves, cubby holes, walls and doorways with the most lavish display of holly, mistletoe, silver gold and red ribbons, Christmas trees, lighting, sparkles, mangers, golden stars and candy canes. Everywhere one looked could be seen the majestic drippings of upscale taste that is the store's trademark.

The store closes early at five p.m. to regular shoppers. Two hours later it re-opens to hundreds of invitation-only guests, the store's most exclusive customers.

It began like any other performance with me seated at the piano and Margaret, Helene and our new member gathered closely around. Margaret turns the keyboard pages while everyone sings along. The others have no need for the black binders from last year as the repertoire has been fully committed to memory. Everything seems much more comfortable this year and because of this, our performances are bolder, filled with greater expression, sung with greater depth.

We sing to the throngs of happy shoppers who mill throughout the crowd with their glossy red Neiman's shopping bags. Well-heeled in their suits and sable coats, they shop and listen while sipping warm cider and chilled Dom Perignon. As is typical, the avid music-lovers are always the first to form in semi-circle around us. They merely listen, nod, sway, hum along, and clap in between pieces. Some sing along quietly while others just listen and smile. Some smile at us as if they know us, their twinkling eyes seemingly wanting to relay some inaudible message. Christmas has returned and beyond all the glitz and glamour and privilege, the underlying glow of the spirit that anticipates the birth of the Savior has returned. The mood is festive and merry.

The first half of our performance breezes through easily, and my fingers are now fully warmed-up. The second half then begins as the four of us begin crooning the words to Silent Night.

As I look into the crowd, I notice two new men who have gathered into the circle of listeners. One of them, the younger man, looks vaguely familiar. My fingers continue to strike the chords, playing the underlying E flat melody. While playing, I continue to study his familiar face, trying to recall the reason for his familiarity. How do I know him? Do I know him? I cannot remember who he is. I do not recall his name. But something about him is definitely familiar.

My gaze then transfers to the older man standing next to him, no doubt his father as the resemblance is uncanny. The elder man holds a red shopping bag in one hand, and his other arm is wrapped around his son. Both appear solemn, somewhat troubled, and yet there is something comforting in the way the father hugs his adult son, holding him tightly at his side. Among this crowd of the merry, these two appear stranded and alone with one holding onto the other for safety.

Without the piano pausing, an easy transition leads into the next carol. My eyes remain focused on the curious pair before me, the son who seems vaguely familiar. *Who is that?* I wonder silently. Who is he? I know him from somewhere, I just can't recall where.

And then, suddenly, it comes to me. The name flashes like a light from the sky across my mind. Miklo. His nickname in high school. I never knew what his real name was. I don't think anyone did. Everyone always called him by his nickname. A year behind me, he was a leader in everything – sports, dating, grades, very popular. The kid who had it all. A boy destined for greatness.

Until the day of the car accident.

I had only heard about it from others, several years ago when it had occurred. The mangled jeep, unrecognizable. The ambulance. I had heard that he was in critical condition for weeks. After that, months in a coma. Unexpectedly, he had suddenly awakened one day in his hospital bed. I was told there had been extensive brain damage and that he could no longer speak. Huge gaps of his memories had been erased from his mind, and he was unable to recall names or recognize his friends. Because of the damage, he had not been able to return to school. Instead, the ensuing years had been spent undergoing grueling workouts with a physical therapist. I had heard that though his condition had improved, he had never quite made a full recovery.

Although I have not seen him since high school, I know for certain that this young man is the very same Miklo. The face is still the same although now it is more handsome, older. The mischievous grin is now replaced with that of seriousness. He is still handsome, and wears dark brown trousers, a button-down shirt and a navy blazer. His gaze has not wavered once from the gleaming marble floor at his feet. Chestnut brown eyes that once sparked so full of life now possess an emptiness, devoid of the shared seasonal spirit of those who surround him. He is now taller than before, his body long and lean, and he stands just a hair above his father standing at his side. It is hard to fathom that it is actually Miklo standing before my very eyes. His vacant eyes do not waver from the polished stone beneath him. He does not see me. He would not recognize me anyway. While he resembles the youth I remember from all the wild keg parties, the reality is that he is not the same, having met a fate that drastically altered his course.

While my fingers continue to play on auto-pilot, my focus is not on the music. I sing in sync with my friends. I sing the memorized lines of the alto part but I do not know what I am singing. I no longer hear the words as my gaze transfers from the son to the father. He is perhaps in his mid-forties but appears much older. The toll taken has prematurely grayed a full head that was once chestnut as is evidenced by the few traces left in its original color. His face also shows too many lines, the signs of one who has suffered too much. He pulls his son closer to him while continuing to clutch the shopping bag at his side. I see that the bag, while opened, is empty. I imagine that he really didn't come here with Miklo to shop. Or perhaps he did. Perhaps he had high hopes of an extravagant shopping trip with his son. But I don't think this was the case. I imagine that it took much effort to get his ill child out of the house in order to place him in a different setting, one that would hopefully induce some kind of spark to this unanimated individual. It is a miracle that he is even alive.

I notice the care he took to dress for tonight's event. A brown tweed jacket mixed with charcoal gray trousers. A dark shirt and a pale red tie. I see the love he has for his boy as he pulls him even closer. The two of them stand together in the midst of all the chaos and listen silently as the music continues.

The girls and I rattle off several more tunes – Hark Hear the Angels Sing, Rudolph, Adestes Fideles – while father and son remain unmoved in the same spot, just listening. The crowd has grown larger as more guests have entered through the red carpet of the valet. The surrounding noise and laughter reaches high into the rafters, so much so that the only way anyone can hear the musical entertainment is if they are directly surrounding us. Several within the circle have already wandered off to do their shopping, to refill their empty flutes. And their spots are instantly replaced with other curious onlookers and music-lovers that stop for a brief respite to soak in the holiday music. The mood is gay, all except for the father and son who remain bonded together like two ships in a storm.

Then, I see something next to the father begin to move. The tiniest flicker of motion. So minute, one would barely notice. My gaze wanders back to the source of this motion, to the son. The movement comes from his lips. Lips that part and begin to form words, singing words. Ever so slightly his lips part and with the barest trace of movement I see that he is mouthing the words to O Little Town of Bethlehem. He whose memory has been all but nearly erased, is now mouthing the words from the faintest portion of a memory that has somehow managed to survive. Because his chest remains still, I realize he is not actually singing out loud. But nonetheless, he is singing. He is remembering.

Simultaneously, his father begins to witness the very same miracle. Holding his son tightly, he stares into the boy's lost expression and sees that the mouth that has not uttered a single word since their arrival has now begun to move. At first he seems confused, as if he is trying to understand what the boy is attempting to communicate. He watches as the formation of words come from the boy's lips. But he quickly realizes that although no sound is audible, his son is indeed mouthing the words to the same ancient holiday carol sung by the choirs at midnight mass. The father's eyes widen as the miracle of this unexpected happening begins to fully materialize in his mind. Somehow the music has reached this wounded young man. Somehow the music has triggered a chord of faint recognition. With a vacant stare, Miklo continues to sing, word for word, the lyrics to the forgotten hymn.

The father cannot hold back the tears that begin to form. His stare moves from that of his son to the floor. He tries to compose himself but cannot, and tears begin to roll down his cheeks as he continues holding his son tightly against him. He does not attempt to wipe them away, and they continue to float silently down his cheeks.

Despite the bustle of our surroundings, all I see is the two of them. My mind has shut out all exterior noise and distractions, and it is if I am on an isolated bend with me on one end and the two of them on the other. I can feel that father's pain. I can see how moved he is that for this brief period in time his son has somehow managed to recapture a glimmer of yesterday. There is the implicit understanding that these rare capsules for them are brief and too far between.

After returning home, I continue thinking about what occurred tonight. And it begins to occur to me that beyond the world in which we pretend to cling to and control so tightly, there is really a truer reality, another realm, the true beauty in which we all live. It is a world in which no one is isolated but rather, all are interconnected either through the conscious or the unconscious. It is one that moves forward, never backward, and depends on all its creatures that live within to keep its rotation in motion. One touches another without ever realizing it, and in doing so helps to create a new awareness, the realization of new possibilities and certainties, and miracles of hope that one could have never before imagined.

I begin to realize that true solitude is not of this world even though it often seems so. Just like my old friend who remains within the confines of a mind shut down, his father makes sure that he is not alone. An old friend from years past who happens to be at the same event and recognizes him although he has no memory of her...one is never alone. Even a failed mind that is unable to recognize his friends or relish in the glories of the past...somehow that mind remembers something that was important, something that meant something, something that can unlock a door. One is never alone.

It begins to dawn on me that, despite all my earlier struggles of believing I was alone in this world, that quite the opposite was true. I was never alone. I was never alone in my anxiety. I was never alone with the overwhelming gray clouds. I was never alone in my secrets. I was never alone in my self-defeating beliefs. I was never alone in my sense of hopelessness. I was never alone. There was always someone who was watching, another who saw, and even more than I gave credit to who cared a great deal.

January 13, 1987
Wt: 104 lbs.

I have been seeing Mister Persistent for a month now. I like him. A lot. I figure better tell him the truth now, and allow him to exit quickly if he chooses. I tell him that I have an eating disorder. Before now, I have never verbalized this statement out loud. I have never uttered this to another soul. I have never admitted fully to another that I have this problem.

He does not appear surprised. He says he knew something was wrong, he just didn't know what. He says that our relationship was never founded upon the cornerstone of my food and weight issue, nor will it ever be. He does not fear things as I always have. Instead, his is a completely different viewpoint. He says the future is much like driving along the back roads of the countryside without a map. Many roads will often lead to the same destination. While the final destination may be the ultimate goal, it is the drive and scenery that matter most.

November 30, 1987
Wt: 106 lbs.

The wedding is in two months. My family still can't believe it because after all, I was the one who always vowed to never marry, to never have children. Now here I stand, eating every word I previously said, even marrying before many of my friends.

I know my mother questions the timing of this huge step. While she does not voice this opinion, I feel her concern as she wonders how my struggles will fare or compete within an infant marriage. In my father's eyes, I see the sadness, the sadness of his eldest daughter to whom he's always been close moving a thousand miles away. I wish my father wasn't so sad. It makes me sad to see him so sad.

No question they are happy for me, happy that *he* makes me so happy, happy that we are all in agreement in my choice of a mate. But still, that *thing* is still there, present, lingering like the smell of smoke after a fire. The unfinished business that has served to scar and deter the path during these past five years. They have yet to witness this great looming mystery solved, the battle won, the illness healed, and therefore my imminent departure bears a bittersweet ring. I know they feel they are sending me out before I am prepared, letting go before they are ready, all without the benefit of having seen the final result – healing – that they've hoped and prayed for. They feel they have not performed well in their roles as parents despite the fact that I have not been a child for some time now, and yet they are having to finally let it all go, to release their burdens and hopes and sadness. I try to assure them that they indeed did well, and also to reinforce just how much I love them and appreciate all they have done for me. Yet I still cannot find words to explain the reasons for my not eating, only that I feel certain it was never meant to punish them, that it was never because of them, that it was not their fault and that it was my own inability to see or correctly handle my own challenges.

Never have I once envisioned a life lived away from my family. The notion seemed inconceivable as nobody, absolutely no one in my family has ever lived outside this city. How odd that I have chosen to do this as I know I am the one viewed as least likely to stand on her own two feet, the one least likely to take a risk of this magnitude, the one who clings the most to family despite the long winding arm's distance. I am the one least likely to move a thousand miles from home, to a city where I know no one and yet, due to that unmistakable inside gut feeling that says *yes this is the correct road to follow*, here I pack my suitcases and my box of saved things while having absolutely no clear vision of what the future holds next year or the year after or a dozen more years down the road.

I am being urged forward by that soft silent voice inside that I have just begun to learn to listen to. Its voice, stilled for so many years and not used to being recognized, bears all the traces of human thought and feeling yet it is invisible, intangible. I ignored this voice for so many years, the voice that was fighting for my ears and heart to pay attention, the voice that urged me to listen, that voice that desired my submission to the insight and knowledge that it had to offer. That voice within, the voice of the soul, went hungry for too long. And now that I have begun to listen to it again, to recognize its value, I realize that this is something that never really went away. Ignored and belittled to the point of starvation, it finally relinquished its battle and succumbed to a deep sleep within the safety and protection of its soul walls where it waited patiently for that spark to once again ignite and thus begin the process of reawakening and emitting its endless supply of energy.

I have never really had to stand on my own two feet, alone in this world without the safety net of my family. And yet didn't I feel utterly alone all those years, alone in my battles, alone in my starvation, alone in my fears and my worries, alone in my doubts that I was a capable human being?

This separation was not always present. I now remember what I have long forgotten, a time when everything felt connected, a connection to everything surrounding me as well as to myself. I was six years old. Eight sets of aunts and uncles, several great-aunts, and dozens of cousins all gathered on Christmas Eve in the warmth of my grandparents' home. The frost and freeze of that late December evening cast an irony against the mood within where a crackling blaze popped and glowed in the living room fireplace, and my grandfather was all smiles while donned with a fake white beard and red hat. Under the tree set hundreds of gifts wrapped in gold and trimmed in red and silver. There were presents for everyone. My great-aunts who always seemed to be joined at the hip and were never without smiles, made the rounds by giving everyone great big bear hugs. And then once they were done, they would begin making the rounds of hugs yet again. With more than forty young cousins in count, all dashing from room to room with boundless energy, the atmosphere was charged, palpable, magical. Indeed everything around me was, at that moment, magical.

I was not the only one who sensed this radiating energy. From her kitchen perch, Alfretta, too, beamed at the chaos while carving the turkey and stirring the oyster dressing. Despite the raucous, my grandparents seemed thoroughly amused with the antics of their growing brood of grandchildren who scampered about recklessly over their velvet gold sofas. It was an uncontainable energy, unstoppable, for reasons I could never explain except to say that it was always there, always present at these family gatherings at my grandparents' home. For no reason at all, all the cousins would hop up and down like bunnies, hour after hour, until it was time to play 'marching human train' again across every piece of their antique furniture.

It was a time when I felt a deep connection to my family, both immediate and extended. Without it being said, it was as if I instinctively knew and trusted this unique place that was mine within the world, my roots as part of this large family that loved me just because. It was a time when anything seemed possible, when any goal had merit and worth, and anything at all could be attained. It was an atmosphere of hope and belonging, and one that was nurtured by love. There was no such thing as fear or "you can't do it" within this large group. Even at that young age, I knew there was something awesome in the fact that my grandparents had raised nine children, built two businesses and maintained a strong faith that served to guide their steps and decision-making. In their minds, nothing was impossible. Everything was possible. Life was a long walk of courage and faith.

Somewhere, somehow, I had forgotten this. I had forgotten that I had ever once felt this way. Somehow I had forgotten that I had once known and believed in this. It was always there, this core, but it had been shoved aside to make room for the negativities and the false beliefs that I taught myself to be true.

There was indeed a time when this connection had been present. And then the separation began to interfere. Interfered with the fears and worries and doubts. Had this separation come from within, or had it been the result of external situations? Perhaps both. Are they not intertwined?

Once the connection was lost, severed, forgotten, and the separation entered, the downward spiral began. And looking back, I see that this did not occur immediately. I ignored the warning signs. I pretended that important things did not matter. I told myself that I did not matter. I convinced myself that what the others had said about me, those things that were not accurate, were indeed true. And I believed the lies. The wall of separation was built slowly and over time, brick by brick, word by word, belief by belief. And once this wall was built, once that last bit of separation had fully constructed, there was no turning back.

No one could see it. No one could see the wall of separation that I had built, the wall that separated me from the real person I was inside.

While I begin to understand a bit more than I did last year and the year before that, there is still much left unexplained, and more that I still do not understand.

Through this man that I am about to marry, I feel I have regained much of that former self that I lost, the part that wants to return, the part that was real but forgotten. I feel none of this separation when I am with him, but rather those austere walls beginning to topple and fall. This is what needs to happen.

We are moving a thousand miles away to start our new life together. While I am excited, there is the underlying terror of the magnitude of this new life. I do not know what the future brings. I do not know how to start fresh in a city and state in which I know no one. I do not know how it will be done but somehow I will find a way.

Although it remains a terrifying challenge, in my mind it does not pose the same crippling torment like it once did. I am just beginning to learn how to make my own decisions, how to realize the many choices available, how to alter a mindset that now sees promise and hope rather than despair. Despite little improvement in my weight, I haven't been as stuck on the idle path of the past but rather, moving forward. And while I still may not be able to vision the exact ending to this chapter, the finale of how this eating situation concludes, I feel somewhat better equipped with the right tools to keep forging ahead.

I am learning to view issues and problems differently, not as forces that bring me down, but rather as challenges in which to overcome. I have a long way to go. I have much to do. There remain many issues with which I must face and deal with, and I will meet each one no matter how long it takes.

I will be fine, and this time I believe that.

January 15, 1988
Wt: 109 lbs.

My wedding is next week. I had another dream. But this was unlike those of the past that represented either a longing for what was not or an outer realm vision relaying a message.

This dream dealt with an issue that needed to be dealt with long ago. And now that I have faced this demon, I know this issue is finally over. It will never hurt me again.

Sleep overcomes my conscious state and transfers me into a world distanced by decades, a place from the past from where I have not ventured back since the age of eight.

I am now a grown woman of twenty-three, and there is still a matter that needs to be dealt with. I am finally ready to deal with it. I need to deal with it before starting my new life at the altar. This issue will not imprison me any longer.

I drive back to the familiar grounds of Amberwild Street, home of my birthplace, the tiny three-bedroom house that sheltered the seven of us until it could budge no further. It is the isolated street off a major thoroughfare where I saw my first snow and where, along with my brothers and sisters, we built our first snowman complete with nose carrot and beach slippers. It is where we gathered tadpoles from the ditch in the late afternoons of the stifling summer months, and placed them along with their polluted water into dirty sand buckets, then sold them door-to-door to our elderly neighbors for ten cents apiece.

It is the street where I got bit by the Doberman pincher that lived in the house across from us, and where I later secretly celebrated his demise after he got hit by a car. It is where we got our first pet, an English cocker spaniel who patiently allowed us to ride her backside as if she were a horse. It is where I religiously studied the Girl Scout manual and labored tirelessly to earn every badge. It is where my mother proudly sewed them onto the green arm band that flanked my uniform.

Amberwild Street was where we all believed in Santa Claus. Even the Tooth Fairy and the Easter Bunny knew our address here. It is where my father strung the Tarzan rope on the tallest limb of the oak tree in the backyard, and where we would swing for hours despite several broken arms, cuts and bruises. It is where we routinely plucked fistfuls of red roses from our next-door neighbor's prized hybrids, and created large bouquets then given to our mother. It is home to the memory of my mother bringing home my youngest brother from the hospital following his birth. Standing expectedly in the driveway with the car was still idling, I reached for the bundle cradled in her arms and explained that from now on I would look after him.

This was the street of my youth, the containment of so many memories of happiness and innocence. And among all of these, one dreadful one, the blight that scarred an otherwise surreal existence here on the grounds of Amberwild Street.

The ebony RX-7 pauses in front of the old house where I grew up. Idling at the curb side, I see that all traces of our youth are now gone. The familiar driveway is absent of tricycles and bicycles and big wheels and plastic swords and medieval shields. There is no longer a half-dozen pair of roller skates left at the front door for someone to trip over. Someone has re-painted the garage door, erasing the rounded dents and dings and blackened scuff marks from that which once served as a tennis backboard. The yard is neat and the St. Augustine is full, and there are no longer any brown dirt patches from the heavy traffic of little feet that once used it as a daily playground. To the right, the garden of rosebushes in our neighbor's side yard remains, and it is now even more fleshed-out with new growth buds and fleshy fauna. Time has continued on but the memories still remain.

I press the accelerator and head further down the street, toward my destination, toward the source of so much pain. At the stop sign, I turn left and drive as if there is no hurry. The homes are painted the same as I remember. The gardens have matured. There is nobody outside except for me. I begin to slow, and then turn into the curb that faces the very last house. I stare at the tiny brick ranch before me. It appears much smaller than I remembered. However, the same 1968 green Chevrolet sedan remains parked at the rear of the driveway, directly in front of the garage door. The paint is peeling and now covered in rust. In fact, as I glance back again at the house, it too bears the same unkempt appearance. Weeds swim alongside the crabgrass overcome by dandelions, and the stark landscape beds are bereft of any plantings. Four picture windows surround the front door, and each is in desperate need of Windex. The drapes are drawn tightly shut. Everything looks entirely deserted and it reminds me of the kind of house that, when we were kids out trick-or-treating, we would have passed over because it didn't look friendly.

I sit in my car and hesitate before finally tossing the keys into my purse. I fight the urge to start the car again and drive off, to drive away and never return. But no, there is business to take care of. And this is the only place where that can be done. I exit the car and slam the door behind me. Beads of dampness from the humidity cling to my forehead as I begin what seems like an interminable walk up the shallow driveway. I'm not even certain whether this family still lives here. The mother is who I have come to see. She is the only one I will deal with. I want to tell her what her son did to me. I want to tell her what her adult son did to an innocent little girl.

I want to let her know the shame her son caused, a shame that cloaked my entire being like an invisible smelly tarp whose odor would not subside no matter how much washing or bathing I did. I want to confront her. I want to ask: How could he do that to me? How could he do that to an eight-year-old girl! I want to tell her about the secret I have carried ever since, a secret I believed would protect me from further harm, yet a secret that only served to protect him.

I want to let her know about the fear that was instilled to an innocent that should have never been introduced to such darkness. I want her to know that until that night, I had never known such fear, and that once the terror entered it never left, and only grew stronger over time, more fearful and violent with each passing year. I want to tell her how ruined I felt, how dirty, how disgusting, and how ashamed I have always felt because of this. I want her to know that it ruined my perception of boys from that point on, making it impossible to trust members of the opposite sex especially after the onset of adolescence. I want to tell her that, with the exception of my father and brothers, I did not trust any males, especially those who showed an interest during the teenage years. I want her to know how much of my life he stole.

I want to lash out at her with all these things. I want to hurt her with the truth. I want to make her understand what he did to me, the ramifications that kept continuing and encircling the older I got. I want to punish this mother. I want her to feel my rage. I want her to suffer.

I want to hash it out, face-to-face, with the mother. But I do not want to tell the son, the perpetrator. I do not ever want to see him again. Although I have not seen him since this single incident that forever changed my life, I wish that his face did not still continue to haunt my memories. I wish that that awful, mocking, jeering face did not continue to haunt, but it does. Much to my disgust, I can still recall what he looked like. I can still smell the odor of sweat upon his skin. To this day, it is a smell that still sickens me.

I want the mother to know all of this, and I want her to pay dearly. I want her to know that her son is the worst kind of human being that exists. I want all of them to pay, his entire family. I want him to die and rot in hell. I want his entire family to rot in hell by their association. I want to spit on their graves.

I want for their house to burn to the ground, leaving no traces of anything they loved behind, turning all they once owned into a smoky heap of burning ashes. I hold all of them responsible. How could he have done that to me? Surely his parents had some idea of what their son was capable of.

My arms tremble as I near the front door. Heavy steps forge along the concrete. Each step weighs a ton as the slow march to the door continues. My eyes focus on the drab front door painted dark brown. I walk nearer and nearer.

I stand on the front porch, a concrete slab that bears no ornamentation, no flower pots, no welcome mat, no door wreath. There is nothing other than windblown traces of top soil from the deserted flower beds below. My palms are sweaty but I am determined, determined to meet this woman again after all these years. I am determined to make her life hell. She will pay for this. Somehow, someone will pay for what he did.

I press the doorbell and step back.

There is no time to change my mind before the door opens. She peers at me through the screen with a dull expression, as if I were an encyclopedia salesman. She looks older than I remembered. Her hair, now fully gray, is pulled back in a tight bun, and thin wisps of hair hang loosely down the sides of her face. She wears an old dress of brown cotton that has never seen an iron and resembles a well-used dishrag. She has grown much older, and is even thinner than I recall. Her forearms are thin and wrinkled and spotted with brown patches. She continues to stare at me in silence, waiting for me to make the first remark.

"Do you remember me?" I choke out the words, inwardly seething at her lack of responsiveness.

She shakes her head no. Beyond her perched stance, I feel the warmth of heat emanating through the living room, pouring through the tiny holes of the screen door to the outside where I stand. Along with the heat comes that odor, that acrid smell of her son, the smell that has created its own little pocket of sickness within my memory where it has remained the unwelcome guest for all these years.

That smell – I step back trying to avoid it but suddenly it is all around me, clinging to my clothes and to the strands of my hair, filling my nostrils with its sickening stench. It is everywhere now — on the threads of my clothing, in my hair, in the pores of my skin, on my shoelaces, mixing with the moisture in my eyes. It envelops me and no matter how many steps I may take backwards, I cannot escape its odor.

Nausea overwhelms me, and I fight the urge to vomit right there on her doorstep. My stomach does flips and everything surrounding me seems to suddenly turn hazy. I feel dizzy. I want to throw up right then and there. My body warns that it will be sick any second. But somehow, I fight this urge. I will not allow it. I will not allow it to overcome and interfere with this mission. His memory will not sicken me any longer. It will no longer defeat me, not after I've come this far, not after I've driven all this way. Not after I've taken the long trek up this hated driveway to this hated doorstep to this hated house where I now stand before this hated mother. No. Nothing, not even the overwhelming stench and sickness will prevent me from saying what I have come here to say.

The taste of bitterness continues to roll across my tongue, an acrid taste that won't go away. At this moment, I feel the absolute blackness of hatred roll through my veins, overpowering my mind, filling out every fiber of my being. Hatred consumes me, overpowering even the sickness I feel. The rage. A rage whose weight is heavier than anything I've ever known before. It is a pure black rage of absolute hatred. I cannot carry this rage any longer. I have carried it for too long. It is time for her to carry it.

I introduce myself. I watch her face as the vague recollections begin forming in her mind, as she travels back in time to more than a decade earlier. She remembers. She remembers that there were five of us: me and my younger brothers and sisters. She remembers as if it is, for her, the vaguest of memories, those most difficult to recollect. It induces neither happiness nor sadness in her demeanor that remains unchanged. She looks old and tired and worn out.

I hate the fact that she mentions my brothers and sisters even though she does not recall them by name. I do not want her to refer to them at all, to somehow invade their privacy and thus possibly tarnish them in the same manner her son tarnished me. I do not want any part of this sick household to touch one hair on the heads of my siblings. Stay away from them, do not mention them, my insides scream in fury.

I struggle for something to lean against as I feel the strength in my knees begin to buckle. However, there is nothing that offers support. I must say what I have come to say, and then get the hell out of here before the hatred and bitterness take over completely, until I am obliterated into a speck of nothingness.

I open my mouth, about to speak, but before the first tormented words can escape, she says matter-of-factly, "My son died. About a year ago it was – he died."

I am so stunned I am unable to speak. Dead? Dead? I am not prepared for this unexpected news. Dead. Dead. It is the last thing I ever expected to hear.

She pronounces it so completely devoid of any emotion that even the undeniable finality of death seems to escape her declaration. It is said with the same emptiness as if I told someone I went to the grocery and bought bananas. My mouth drops, and I don't know how to respond.

As I continue staring at her through the aluminum screen, I begin to notice now much shorter she is and how much older she looks than from my earlier first impression. It begins to dawn on me just how careless her appearance actually is. This is a woman who no longer cares about anything. Looking beyond her, I see through the dim shadows of the living room that old sheets cover the furniture and newspapers are strewn across an unswept floor. There is no care here. This is a woman who no longer cares about anything. Not about her appearance. Not about her home. Not about anything. I look closer into her face and see there are many more lines and creases than what I first observed. Her gray eyes are watery and yellowed in the corners. I begin to realize that staring before me is the face of a woman who has suffered greatly. This is a woman who lives with suffering, and who does not escape it during any time of any day. Staring back at me, beyond the blankness, is the unmistakable face of grief.

I think to myself, she has suffered enough. I know that I cannot tell her what I came here to say. I cannot do it. She has already paid, and continues to pay each day. I feel the dark thoughts begin to melt away, all the feelings of anger and rage as they begin to slowly wash out of me along with the incurring debts of shame and guilt, and the black fury of hatred. They are all rolled into one just as they have always been, but there is no longer any need to continue to carry them with me. For now, they need to be discarded. And they will be left here, right here on this doorstep, after she closes the door. I will leave it here. I will not take it back with me. I will deposit it here where it will then be scattered by the wind in all directions until there are no traces left. She will never know, and I no longer feel the need to hurl my stones at her.

There is no one left to punish, not even myself. She will never know the truth, and for me, that is okay. It is over. It is finally over.

I offer no condolences, and say nothing further. It is over and there is no need to speak. There is nothing left to say. It is over.

In silence, I turn and head back to the car. I start the engine, press my foot on the accelerator, and leave Amberwild Street for good.

www.ingramcontent.com/pod-product-compliance
Lightning Source LLC
Chambersburg PA
CBHW060457290526
45791CB00001B/152